Aids to ENT

CW00381799

Aids to ENT

Victoria Moore-Gillon
BSc(Hons)   FRCS   FRCS(Ed)

Senior Registrar, The Royal National
Throat, Nose and Ear Hospital, London

Nicholas Stafford
MB   ChB   FRCS

Senior Registrar, ENT Department,
St Mary's Hospital, London

CHURCHILL LIVINGSTONE
EDINBURGH LONDON MELBOURNE AND NEW YORK 1987

CHURCHILL LIVINGSTONE
Medical Division of Longman Group UK Limited

Distributed in the United States of America by
Churchill Livingstone Inc., 1560 Broadway,
New York, N.Y. 10036, and by associated
companies, branches and representatives
throughout the world.

First published 1987

ISBN   0-443-03270-X

British Library Cataloguing in Publication Data
Moore-Gillon, Victoria
   Aids to ENT. — (Aids).
   1. Otolaryngology
   I. Title   II. Stafford, Nicholas
   617'.51   RF46

Library of Congress Cataloging in Publication Data
Moore-Gillon, Victoria.
   Aids to ENT.

   1. Otolaryngology — Outlines, syllabi, etc.
I. Stafford, Nicholas.   II. Title.   [DNLM:
1. Otolaryngology — outlines.   WV 18 M822a]
RF58.M66   1987   617'.51'00202   87-8006

Produced by Longman Singapore Publishers (Pte) Ltd
Printed in Singapore

Preface

Undergraduate students and ENT surgeons starting their training find themselves confronted by so many new clinical conditions and so much new information that a list can help rapidly organise and clarify matters in a way that an ordinary textbook might not. Those with a little more experience — in hospital or general practice — find lists useful as a prompter for the memory when confronted with an uncommon problem, a symptom resistant to simple explanation, or an impending examination. Learning from lists — particularly other people's lists — is not a substitute for clinical experience, personal teaching and the reading of textbooks; the examination candidate relying solely on cramming lists of facts may come spectacularly unstuck. This book supplements and does *not* replace patient contact and the excellent conventional textbooks of ENT available.

Useful lists are always a compromise since completeness and clarity are all too easily inversely related. Even a consistent and systematic approach throughout may hinder rather than help by occasionally relegating the commonest cause to the most obscure corner. We have organised this book largely according to the symptoms with which the patient may present. We have steered a middle course as far as is possible, but inevitably some aspects of ENT are dealt with in greater detail than others. There is more here than the undergraduate student *has* to know, but much that we hope he or she will *want* to know. Postgraduate examination candidates will find that most, but not all, of the topics we have included are covered in sufficient breadth (but naturally not depth) for their needs.

London, 1987
V. M.-G.
N. S.

Contents

PART ONE

The ear

Anatomy

EMBRYOLOGY

1. External ear
    (i) The pinna is derived from first and second branchial arch mesenchyme

    (ii) The external auditory canal is derived from the first branchial cleft

2. Middle ear
    (i) The first branchial pouch (tubotympanic recess) becomes the Eustachian tube and middle ear cleft. First arch mesenchyme forms the middle, fibrous, layer of the tympanic membrane, the malleus and the incus. The stapes develops from second branchial arch mesenchyme

    (ii) Mastoid pneumatisation — Types — Cellular (80%)
                                                      Diploic
                                                      Sclerotic

    (iii) Theories of deficient mastoid pneumatisation —
           Failure of middle ear cleft aeration (Tumarkin)
           Infantile otitis media (Wittmaark)
           Congenital variant (Diamant)

3. Inner ear
The membranous labyrinth is derived from the otic vesicle, which develops from an invagination of ectoderm in the region of the hindbrain

EXTERNAL AUDITORY CANAL

1. 25 mm long in the adult
2. Cartilagenous in its lateral third
3. Bony in its medial two-thirds
4. Lined by keratinising stratified squamous epithelium which also covers the lateral surface of the tympanic membrane
5. No skin adenexae in the medial two-thirds

6. Wax formed from the secretions of the ceruminous glands (modified sweat glands) and sebaceous glands in the cartilagenous portion

MIDDLE EAR CLEFT

1. In the adult the tympanic cavity is a biconcave disc approximately 14 mm in diameter. At its narrowest, the disc is only 2 mm wide
2. Mucosal folds and ossicular ligaments support the ossicles and divide the cleft into several compartments
3. Most of the cleft is lined by a simple non-ciliated cuboidal epithelium
4. The epitympanum, or attic, is that part of the cleft lying above the upper margin of the tympanic membrane
5. The mesotympanum is that part lying directly medial to the tympanic membrane
6. The hypotympanum is that part of the cleft lying below the lower margin of the tympanic membrane

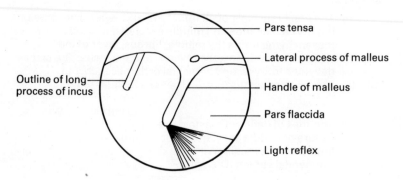

Fig. 1 Otoscopic appearance of right tympanic membrane

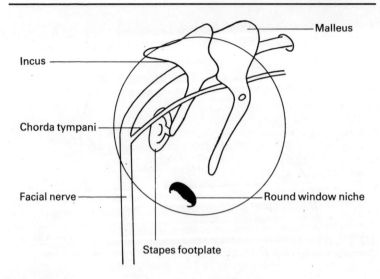

Fig. 2 Position of ossicles in the right middle ear cleft

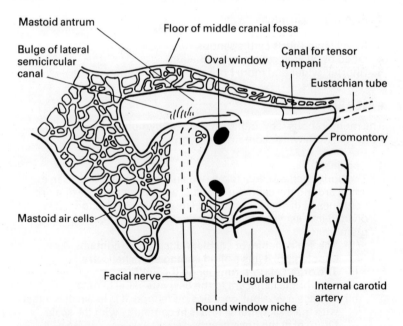

Fig. 3 A sagittal section throught the right middle ear cleft showing the features of the medial wall. The ossicles have been removed

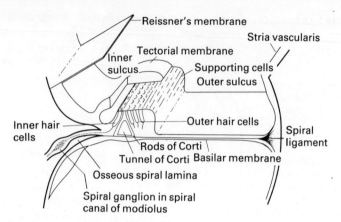

Fig. 4 Transverse section across the scala media and organ of Corti. Part of Reissner's membrane and the tectorial membrane have been removed

EUSTACHIAN TUBE

1. 37 mm long in adults
2. Lateral one-third bony
3. Medial two-thirds cartilagenous
4. Lined by ciliated columnar epithelium
5. Shorter, wider and more horizontal in children

INNER EAR

The membranous labyrinth contains endolymph and lies within the bony labyrinth which contains perilymph

1. Cochlea

The bony cochlea canal takes two and three-quarter turns in a spiral around the central modiolus, which contains the first order neurones of the cochlear nerve. The canal is 35 mm long. It is divided into sections by Reissner's membrane and the basilar membrane:

(i) The scala media, or cochlear duct, which contains endolymph. It has a blind ending at the helicotrema
(ii) The organ of Corti runs along the entire length of the basilar membrane, adjacent to the osseous spiral lamina
(iii) The scala vestibuli contains perilymph. It is in direct contact with the oval window and is in continuity with the scala tympani at the helicotrema
(iv) The scala tympani, which is in direct contact with the round window

Table 1 Organ of Corti hair cells

	Number of rows of cells	Pattern of cilia on hair cell	Share of afferent nerve fibre supply (%)
Inner hair cells	1	2 straight rows	95
Outer hair cells	3–4	3 rows in a W	5

2. Vestibular labyrinth

(i) The membranous semicircular ducts communicate directly with the utricle. The utricle communicates indirectly with the saccule and cochlear duct via the endolymphatic duct. There are three semicircular canals in each labyrinth:
(a) Lateral
(b) Superior
(c) Posterior
The three canals lie at 90° to each other. The two lateral canals lie in the same plane, as does the superior canal of one side and the posterior canal of the opposite side
Each bony canal is locally dilated at one end. This site is known as the ampulla and contains the crista

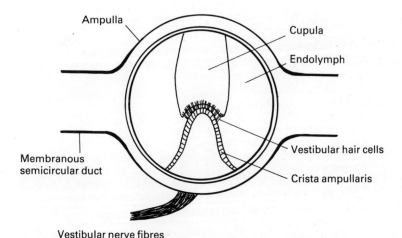

Fig. 5 Section through the ampulla of a membranous semicircular canal

The cupula is a gelatinous mass which acts as a valve across the ampulla. It is attached to the duct wall opposite the crista. The cilia of the crista hair cells enter the substance of the cupula

(ii) The utricle and saccule also contain areas of specialised sensory epithelium, the maculae. The macula of the utricle lies in the horizontal plane, that of the saccule in the vertical plane

The maculae are flat structures with ciliated cells and supporting cells very similar to those of the cristae. The hair cell cilia project into the gelatinous otolithic membrane on the surface of which are the otoconia

The blood supply to the inner ear comes from the internal auditory artery, an end artery branch of the anterior inferior cerebellar artery. Venous drainage is into the petrosal and sigmoid sinuses

Physiology

HEARING

1. The function of the middle ear is to match the acoustic impedances of air and perilymph so that loss of sound energy at the oval window interface is kept to a minimum. This is achieved by:
   (i) The ossicular lever system
   (ii) The tympanic membrane/oval window hydraulic system
2. The function of the inner ear is to convert mechanical into electrical energy. This is brought about by the hair cells of the organ of Corti. Movement of the stapes footplate in the oval window produces vibrations in the perilymph of the scala vestibuli and scala tympani. Basilar membrane movement follows in the form of a travelling wave which begins at the basal end of the membrane and reaches a point of maximum membrane displacement at a point which is frequency dependent. The wave then quickly fades. Displacement of the basilar membrane produces shearing forces between the tectorial membrane and hair cell cilia. Movement of hair cell cilia is accompanied by electrical activity in the cells afferent nerve fibres
3. The central connections of the cochlear nerves are the cochlear nuclei in the medulla. The site of the auditory cortex is the superior temporal gyrus

BALANCE

1. The function of the vestibular labyrinth is to monitor the position and movement of the body in relation to its environment. Whilst the semicircular canal cristae sense angular acceleration the maculae of the utricles sense gravitational tilt and linear acceleration
2. The function of the saccular maculae remains uncertain
3. The vestibular hair cells are directionally polarised. On each cell a single kinocilium is localised to one side of the bundle of stereocilia. The kinocilia of each crista all lie in one direction:

either towards or away from the adjacent utricle, depending on the canal

4. On the maculae the kinocilia all point towards the linea alba, which is a line running across the centre of each macula

5. Rotational acceleration produces movement of the semicircular canal endolymph in relation to the crista. The resulting movement of the cupula causes distortion of the hair cell cilia of the crista and either a rise or a fall in the neural discharge from the ampulla. There is a corresponding, but opposite, change in the discharge from the ampulla of the contralateral paired canal. Unless the rotation is in the exact plane of one pair of canals then two or all three pairs will be stimulated. Both lateral canals lie in the same plane. Each superior canal lies in the same plane as the contralateral posterior canal

6. Gravitational tilt or linear acceleration produces movement of utricular endolymph in relation to the utricular maculae. Displacement of the otolithic membrane results in hair cell cilia distortion and either a rise or a fall in neural discharge from the maculae (like the semicircular canals, the maculae discharge tonically at rest)

7. The central connections of each vestibular nerve are the vestibular nuclei in the upper medulla and lower pons. The central pathways from the nuclei are:
    (i) The vestibulospinal tract (control of muscle tone)
    (ii) The medial longitudinal bundle to the III, IV and VI nerve nuclei (control of eye movement)
    (iii) The vestibulo-cerebellar tracts (control of coordination and adjustment of movement)

Radiology

CONVENTIONAL RADIOLOGY

1. **Lateral oblique view (Stockholm B)**
   - (i) Mastoid antrum and air cell system
   - (ii) Level of middle cranial fossa dura
   - (iii) Position of lateral sinus

2. **Postero-anterior oblique view (Stenvers)**
   - (i) Internal auditory meatus
   - (ii) Cochlea and semicircular canals
   - (iii) Mastoid process
   - (iv) Petrous apex

3. **25–35° Fronto-occipital view (Townes)**
   - (i) Internal auditory meatus
   - (ii) Cochlea and semicircular canals
   - (iii) Middle ear and bony external meatus

4. **Submento-vertical view**
   - (i) Skull base
   - (ii) Petrous apex
   - (iii) Cochlea and semicircular canals
   - (iv) Mastoid air cell system

TOMOGRAPHY

   - (i) Fractures
   - (ii) Bony destruction
   - (iii) Specific structures
     - a. Internal auditory meatus
     - b. Middle ear and ossicles
     - c. Inner ear
     - d. Jugular fossa

CT SCAN
Tumours

CAROTID ARTERIOGRAPHY
Glomus tympanicum/jugulare

Audiology

CLINICAL ASSESSMENT OF HEARING

1. In children

Table 2 Clinical assessment of hearing in children

Technique	Age group
Reflex tests	0–6 months
Distraction tests	6 months–1 year
Behavioural tests	2–4 years
Conditioned audiometry	4 years +

2. In adults

(i) *Voice perception tests (performed with the non-test ear masked)*
   a. If whispered voice is heard 3 feet from the ear, then the hearing threshold is less than 30 dB
   b. If conversational voice is heard 3 feet from the ear, then the hearing threshold is less than 60 dB

(ii) *Tuning fork tests (512 Hz)*
   a. Rinne test — The Rinne test is positive when air conducted sound (with the struck tuning fork held 6 inches away from the test ear) is heard for a longer duration than bone conducted sound (with the base of the struck tuning fork held on the mastoid process)
   A positive Rinne indicates either normal hearing or a sensorineural loss
   The Rinne test is negative when bone conducted sound is heard for a longer duration than air conducted sound
   A negative Rinne indicates either a conductive hearing loss or a dead ear. If the fork is no longer heard by bone conduction when the non-test ear is masked using a

Barany noise box then the test ear is dead (false negative Rinne)
b. Weber test — If the struck tuning fork is placed firmly on the forehead in the midline then it will be heard in the right ear if there is a conductive hearing loss on that side or a sensori-neural loss in the other ear
If it is heard centrally then the hearing is normal, symmetrically impaired, or there is little difference between the two ears

SUBJECTIVE AUDIOMETRY

1. Pure tone audiometry
(i) To avoid cross-over of sound to the non-test ear this ear must be masked whenever bone conduction thresholds are being assessed
(ii) Masking must also be used when air conduction thresholds are being assessed and there is a difference of more than 45 dB between the thresholds of the two sides

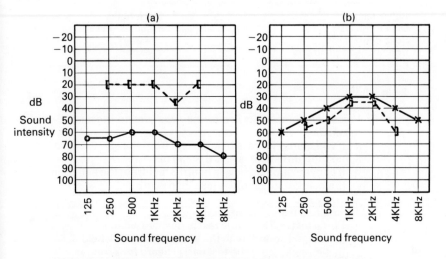

Fig. 6 (a) Otosclerosis: there is a conductive hearing loss with a characteristic Cahart's notch at 2000 Hz in the bone conduction.
(b) Menière's disease: in the early stages of the disease there is a sensory loss predominantly affecting the lower frequencies

2. Speech audiometry

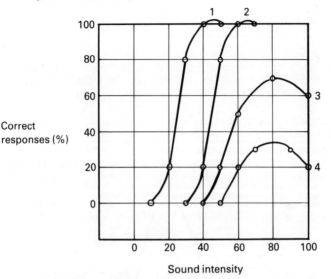

Fig. 7 1 = normal hearing; 2 = conductive hearing loss; 3 = sensory (cochlear) hearing loss; 4 = neural (retrocochlear) hearing loss.

- (i) Optimum discrimination score (ODS) = the maximum percent correct score
- (ii) Speech reception threshold (SRT) = the lowest sound intensity at which the patient achieves a 50% correct response

3. Tests of recruitment
- (i) Alternate binaural loudness balance test
- (ii) Loudness discomfort levels
- (iii) Short increment sensitivity index
- (iv) Difference limen test

4. Tests of adaptation
- (i) Tone decay test
- (ii) Bekesy audiometry
  This provides a combines assessment of hearing threshold, recruitment and adaptation in one test
  Five types of Bekesy audiogram are recognised (Jerger)
  type 1 = normal
  type 2 = sensory hearing loss
  type 3 = neural hearing loss
  type 4 = neural hearing loss
  type 5 = non-organic hearing loss

OBJECTIVE AUDIOMETRY

1. Impedance audiometry

(i) *Tympanometry*

The tympanic membrane functions optimally (when its compliance is maximum) when the pressures on either side of it aré equal. The middle ear cleft pressure, and tympanic membrane compliance, can be assessed by measuring the proportion of a 220 Hz signal that is reflected by the tympanic membrane at different external auditory canal pressures

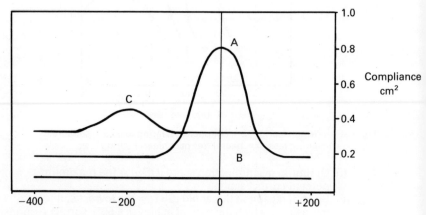

External canal air pressure (mm H$_2$O)

Fig. 8 Type A curve = normal middle ear pressure (average compliance 0.6 cm^2); type B curve = flat tympanogram indicates a middle ear effusion; type C curve = negative middle ear pressure indicates Eustachian tube dysfunction without middle ear effusion

(ii) *Acoustic reflex measurement*

Contraction of the stapedius muscle normally occurs in response to sound 70–100 dB above the hearing threshold. The reflex can be detected as a change in tympanic membrane compliance. It is absent if there is a conductive or a severe neural hearing loss, or in certain types of facial palsy

2. Evoked response audiometry

(i) Electrocochleography (ECoG)
Measurement of electrical activity in the cochlea in response to sound stimulation has two clinical uses
a. Assessment of hearing threshold
b. Diagnosis of certain sensory and neural hearing losses (e.g. Menieres disease, acoustic neuroma)

(ii) Brainstem evoked responses (BSER)
Useful for
a. Assessment of hearing threshold
b. Diagnosis of the site of a neural deafness

(iii) Cortical evoked responses (CER)

Deafness

6000 children in ordinary schools wear hearing aids and another
3500 attend special schools or training units

CAUSES

1. Congenital

    (i) Conductive
        a. Syndrome-related — e.g. Treacher Collins
        b. Isolated — Otosclerosis
                    Ossicular defects
                    Meatal atresia

    (ii) Sensorineural
        a. Genetic — Syndrome-related — e.g. Pendred's
                    — Chromosomal — e.g. Trisomy 18
                    — Isolated — Familial progressive
                                  sensorineural deafness
                                  Inner ear aplasia
                                  Congenital cholesteatoma
        b. Intrauterine — Infective — Rubella
                                  Syphilis
                                  Toxoplasmosis
                                  Cytomegalovirus
                    — Toxins — Hypoxia
                                Kernicterus
                                Drugs
        c. Perinatal — Birth injury
                    Hypoxia/anoxia

2. Acquired

    (i) Conductive
      a. Traumatic — Barotrauma
                Head Injury
                Iatrogenic
      b. Neoplastic — Benign — Osteoma
                      Malignant — SCCa middle ear
      c. Infective — Otitis externa
                Acute suppurative otitis media
                Chronic suppurative otitis media
                Tuberculosis
      d. Miscellaneous — Wax
                    Keratosis obturans
                    Middle ear effusion

    (ii) Sensorineural
      a. Traumatic — Head injury
                Noise
                Iatrogenic
      b. Neoplastic — Benign — Acoustic neuroma
                    — Malignant — SCCa middle ear
      c. Infective — Measles
                Mumps
                Influenza
                Syphilis
                Suppurative labyrinthitis
                Herpes zoster oticus
      d. Degenerative— Presbyacusis
      e. Metabolic — Menière's disease
      f. Toxins — Ototoxic drugs
      g. Vascular — Cardiac bypass surgery
      h. Miscellaneous — In association with other systemic
                    disease (eg diabetes mellitus)
                    Idiopathic

INVESTIGATIONS

1. History
    (i) Onset
    (ii) Duration
    (iii) Progression
    (iv) Otalgia
    (v) Otorrhoea
    (vi) Vertigo
    (vii) Tinnitus
    (viii) Ear disease in childhood
    (ix) Obstetric and neonatal history

    (x) Family history
   (xi) Noise exposure
   (xii) Ototoxic drugs
  (xiii) Trauma

2. Examination
    (i) Ears
   (ii) Nose
  (iii) Neurological

3. Investigations
    (i) Haematology
       a. FBC + ESR
       b. VDRL / TPHA
       c. Blood sugar
       d. Triglycerides
       e. Thyroid function studies
   (ii) Radiology
       a. Mastoid X-rays
       b. Middle ear tomography
       c. Internal auditory meatus X-rays
       d. Temporal bone tomography
       e. CT scan
       f. NMR scan
       g. Sinus X-ray
  (iii) Audiology
       a. PTA
       b. Speech audiometry
       c. Tympanometry, acoustic reflexes and reflex decays
       d. Loudness balance
       e. Tone decay
       f. Bekesy
       g. Evoked response audiometry
       h. Vestibular function studies — Fitzgerald-Hallpike caloric test

The choice of investigations is determined by the clinical findings

EUSTACHIAN TUBE DYSFUNCTION

1. Causes of Eustachian tube obstruction or dysfunction
    (i) Congenital
       a. Absent Eustachian tube, eg Treacher Collins syndrome
       b. Cleft palate
       c. Eustachian tube diverticulae
   (ii) Acquired
       a. Acute salpingitis eg. viral, bacterial, chlorinated water
       b. Chronic upper aerodigestive tract infection

c. Chronic salpingitis
d. Adenoid hypertrophy
e. Allergy
f. Neoplastic eg. nasopharyngeal carcinoma, juvenile angiofibroma
g. Trauma eg barotrauma, post adenoidectomy scarring, irradiation
h. Foreign body
i. Nasal polyps

Obstruction of tubal lymphatics, rather than direct obstruction of the tube, may be the cause of a middle ear effusion in some cases

In one study of 704 4-year-old children a middle ear effusion was present in 20% of them

Table 3 Types of middle ear effusion

Serous fluid (Acute or chronic serous otitis media)	Sterile, low viscosity straw-coloured fluid. Usually associated with an acute history eg common cold, barotrauma. Occasionally CSF following temporal bone fracture with intact TM
Mucoid fluid ('Glue ear')	High viscosity, yellow/grey 'glue' which is commonly sterile on culture. Usually associated with longstanding Eustachian tube dysfunction
Bloody fluid	Usually due to barotrauma, chronic serous otitis media or cholesterol granuloma. More rarely associated with temporal bone fracture, glomus tumour or bleeding tendency
Purulent fluid	The pre-suppurative stage of acute suppurative otitis media

2. **Sequelae of chronic middle ear effusion (usually 'glue ear')**
   (i) Atrophic tympanic membrane
   (ii) Tympanosclerosis
   (iii) Cholesteatoma
   (iv) Ossicular erosion
   (v) Cholesterol granuloma
   (vi) Adhesive otitis media

GLUE EAR IS THE MOST COMMON CAUSE OF DEAFNESS IN CHILDREN

OTOSCLEROSIS

A primary disease of the labyrinthine capsule in which areas of new bone formation can cause fixation of the stapes footplate and a conductive hearing loss. Cochlear involvement with a sensorineural hearing loss may also occur

1. Clinical features
    (i) 90% cases present between the ages of 15 and 45 years
    (ii) Affects 1 in 200 of the Caucasian population
    (iii) Family history in 70%
    (iv) Bilateral in 75%
    (v) Tinnitus in 80%
    (vi) Positional vertigo in 25%
    (vii) Carharts notch in 33%
    (viii) Tympanic membrane usually normal in appearance. Schwartze's sign in 2%
    (ix) Paracusis in 80%

2. Differential diagnosis
    (i) Other causes of ossicular immobility
      a. Congenital fixation of one ossicle
      b. Tympanosclerosis
      c. Chronic secretory otitis media
      d. Chronic adhesive otitis media
    (ii) Ossicular discontinuity
      a. Congenital absence of one ossicle
      b. Traumatic disruption of ossicular chain
      c. Inflammatory ossicular erosion
    (iii) Other bone diseases
      a. Pagets disease
      b. Osteogenesis imperfecta

PRESBYACUSIS

Presbyacusis is a characteristically bilateral sensorineural hearing loss caused by age dependant degenerative changes in the cochlea and its central connections

There are large variations in the individual patients susceptibility to presbyacusis.

Table 4 Types of presbyacusis (after Schuknecht)

	Lesion	PTA	Speech discrimination
Sensory	Degenerative changes in the Organ of Corti	High frequency sensorineural loss	Little impairment
Neural	Loss of neurons in the cochlea and its central connections	Mild sensorineural loss	Severe impairment
Metabolic	Atrophy of the stria vascularis	Characteristically 'flat' loss	Remains relatively good
Mechanical	Impairment of the elasticity of the basilar membrane	High frequency sensorineural loss	Remains relatively good

A combination of two or more of these lesions can coexist

PRESBYACUSIS IS THE MOST COMMON CAUSE OF DEAFNESS IN
ADULTS

ACOUSTIC NEUROMA

Acoustic neuromas comprise 80% of all cerebellopontine angle
tumours and 10% of all brain tumours

Clinical features
  (i) Very rarely present before the age of 30 years
 (ii) Usually present with hearing loss which is sudden in onset in
      5%
(iii) Tinnitus common
 (iv) Unsteadiness occurs in 80%, true vertigo in 33%
  (v) As the neuroma enlarges the otological phase progresses into
      the neurological phase with cranial nerve palsies (V, VII, IX, X,
      XI and XII) and cerebellar dysfunction: finally, symptoms and
      signs of raised intracranial pressure develop
 (vi) Audiological tests characteristically show a retrocochlear type
      of sensorineural hearing loss, although a cochlear type loss
      may occur early on
(vii) Caloric tests show a decreased or absent response from the
      affected side in 95%
(viii) An air contrast CT scan of the internal meatus is virtually
      diagnostic. Brainstem evoked response audiometry shows
      characteristic changes

> In the presence of a unilateral sensorineural hearing loss and an abnormal ipsilateral caloric response an acoustic neuroma must be excluded

SUDDEN SENSORINEURAL HEARING LOSS

A Sensorineural deafness that develops over a period of a few hours or a few days

1. Causes
   (i) Viral infection, e.g. mumps, measles, *Herpes zoster*
   (ii) Vascular, e.g. fat emboli, cardiac surgery
   (iii) Traumatic, e.g. post stapedectomy, noise induced, blunt head injury, labyrinthine membrane rupture
   (iv) Ototoxic drugs
   (v) Labyrinthitis, e.g. secondary to CSOM, syphilis
   (vi) Acoustic neuroma
   (vii) Menières disease
   (viii) Non-organic hearing loss

In two-thirds of patients with a sudden sensorineural hearing loss an identifiable cause is never found

2. Clinical features
   (i) Most cases are unilateral
   (ii) Tinnitus common
   (iii) Vertigo: mild and transient in 40%, severe in 10%
   (iv) Concurrent upper respiratory tract infection in 20%
   (v) PTA appearance variable. A low frequency loss carries the best prognosis

One-third of patients have a return of normal hearing
One-third are left with a 40-80 dB sensorineural loss
One-third have no useful hearing in the ear

A deafness of very sudden onset associated with vertigo carries the worst prognosis.

NOISE TRAUMA

Noise is the second most common cause of sensorineural hearing loss

1. Clinical types
   (i) Noise induced hearing loss
      a. Follows longterm exposure to moderately loud noise (85–95 dB)
      b. Prolonged exposure changes a temporary threshold shift into a premanent threshold shift
      c. The PTA loss characteristically shows a notch at 4 KHz (Boilermakers notch)
      d. Can be an industrial disease
   (ii) Acoustic trauma
      a. Follows short term exposure to an intense noise
      b. The PTA shows a severe high frequency loss which is immediate and permanent
   (iii) Blast trauma
      a. The positive pressure component causes middle ear damage (e.g. tympanic membrane perforation) whilst the negative pressure wave which follows causes damage to the cochlea
      b. Partial recovery of the sensorineural loss can be expected in many cases

DEAFNESS ASSOCIATED WITH SYSTEMIC DISEASE

Causes
   (i) Metabolic
      a. Diabetes mellitus
      b. Myxoedema
      c. Hyperlipidaemia
      d. Paget's disease (may also cause a conductive hearing loss)
   (ii) Inflammatory diseases
      a. Auto-immune diseases — Wegener's granuloma
                             — Cogan's syndrome
      b. Sarcoidosis
   (iii) Neurological diseases — Multiple sclerosis

NON-ORGANIC HEARING LOSS

Non-organic hearing loss is an apparent hearing loss which cannot be attributed to any organic aetiology or structural change within the ear

50% of all patients with a non-organic loss do have a degree of organic hearing loss as well

Detection
   (i) Suspicion on clinical assessment
  (ii) Variations of more than 10 dB on repeating the PTA
 (iii) The PTA fails to show a shadow curve in the normal ear when a
       total hearing loss is claimed in the tested, abnormal ear
 (iv) Positive Stenger test (tuning fork and audiometric)
  (v) Acoustic reflex threshold elicited at a sound intensity below
       the apparent hearing threshold
 (vi) The SPAR test (sensitivity prediction from the acoustic reflex)
 (vii) Bekesy audiometry will often show a type V curve
(viii) Positive delayed speech feedback test
 (ix) Brainstem and cortical evoked response audiometry

AUDITORY REHABILITATION

Deaf children will require oral training as well as auditory training

1. Hearing aids
These can be electrical or non electrical (eg the ear trumpet)

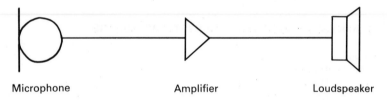

Microphone   Amplifier   Loudspeaker

Fig. 9 Electrical aid

    (i) Requirements of an electrical aid
       a. Adequate amplification of sound input
       b. Control of the volume of sound output, with limitation of
          excessively loud noises which can cause discomfort and
          noise damage to the cochlea, especially in the presence
          of a recuiting deafness
   (ii) Types of electrical aids
       a. Individual aids — Air conducting — Body worn
                                   Behind ear
                                     Spectacle worn
                   Bone conducting — Headworn
       b. Speech training hearing aids — Radio hearing aids
                                        Induction loop aids
                                         Group aids with central
                                         console

2. Family guidance

3. Educational considerations
  (i) Schooling
    a. Grade I — Child wears hearing aid and attends normal school
    b. Grade II — Child attends a partially hearing unit in a normal school
    c. Grade III — Child attends a special centre for the deaf, which may be a residential or day school
  (ii) Sign language
  Severely deaf children may require an alternate means of communication
  There are two basic types of sign language –
  a. Phonetic alphabet
  b. Sign systems (eg British, Paget-Gorman)

Otalgia

PAIN IN THE EAR

CAUSES

1. Local
    (i) External ear
        a. Infective — Perichondritis
                      Otitis externa
                      Bullous myringitis
                      Herpes zoster oticus
        b. Traumatic — Subperichondrial haematoma
                        Instrumentation
        c. Neoplastic — Benign tumours — Osteoma
                        Malignant tumours — Squamous
                        carcinoma
        d. Miscellaneous — Impacted wax
                        — Keratosis obturans
   (ii) Middle ear, mastoid and temporal bone
        a. Infective — Eustachian tube obstruction
                      Acute suppurative otitis media
                      Secretory otitis media
                      Acute mastoiditis
                      Chronic suppurative otitis media
        b. Traumatic — Barotrauma
                      Head injury
        c. Neoplastic — Benign tumours — Acoustic neuroma
                      Malignant tumours — Squamous
                      carcinoma
        d. Miscellaneous — Bell's palsy

2. Referred
    (i) Oral cavity and oropharynx
        a. Dental — Root abscess
        b. Tongue — Carcinoma
        c. Tonsil — Acute tonsillitis
   (ii) Larynx and hypopharynx
        a. Carcinoma

 (iii) Neck
   a. Cervical spine arthritis
   b. Postauricular lymphadenitis
 (iv) Mediastinum — Oesophageal foreign body
  (v) Miscellaneous
   a. Sinusitis
   b. Temporomandibular joint dysfunction

INVESTIGATIONS

1. History
   (i) Onset
   (ii) Duration
  (iii) Progressive
  (iv) Otorrhoea
   (v) Hearing loss
  (vi) Vertigo
  (vii) Recent URTI
 (viii) Trauma

2. Examination
   (i) Pyrexia
   (ii) Ears
  (iii) Nose
  (iv) Oropharynx and oral cavity
   (v) Larynx and hypopharynx
  (vi) Facial nerve function
  (vii) Neck

3. Investigations
   (i) Haematology
    a. FBC + ESR
    b. Blood sugar
   (ii) Radiology
    a. Mastoid X-rays
    b. Paranasal sinus X-rays
    c. Cervical spine X-rays
    d. Orthopantomogram
    e. Temporomandibular joint X-rays
  (iii) Bacteriology — Aural swab
  (iv) Audiometry
    a. PTA
    b. Tympanometry
   (v) Surgical — Biopsy

The choice of investigations is determined by the clinical findings

OTITIS EXTERNA

Causes
(i) Infective
  a. Bacterial — Diffuse otitis externa
                 Furunculosis
                 Malignant otitis externa

Table 5 Furunculosis versus acute mastoiditis

	Furunculosis	Acute mastoiditis
History	Sudden onset of pain	Increase in pain following recent history of otitis media
Examination	Apyrexial No systemic upset TM normal, if visible	Pyrexial General malaise TM shows evidence of otitis media
	Maximum tenderness on palpation of tragus	Maximum tenderness over MacEwen's triangle and mastoid air cells
	Postauricular sulcus absent	Postauricular sulcus intact
Investigations	WBC normal PTA normal or shows a 10–15 dB conductive loss Lateral mastoid X-rays may show air cell clouding due to postauricular soft tissue oedema but SMV view will show a normal air cell system	WBC raised PTA shows a 30–40 dB conductive loss All mastoid X-ray views show clouding or loss of mastoid air cell system
Treatment	Glycerin/ichthammol wick Systemic antibiotics Incision and drainage occasionally required	If the condition is seen before an abscess has developed then a 24-hour trial of parenteral antibiotics is given. Cortical mastoidectomy is undertaken immediately if a mastoid abscess has formed or after 24 hours if there is not a rapid response to antibiotics

   b. Viral — Bullous myringitis
            Herpes zoster oticus (Ramsay Hunt syndrome)
            Herpes simplex
   c. Fungal — *Candida albicans*
            Aspergillus niger
(ii) Non-infective
   a. Localised — Allergy (to topical antibiotics)
            Irradiation
   b. Generalised dermatological disease — Eczema
                              Psoriasis
                              Seborrhoeic otitis
                              externa

MALIGNANT OTITIS EXTERNA

1. Clinical features
   (i) Occurs in elderly diabetics or immunologically
        compromised patients
   (ii) *Pseudomonas pyocyaneus* isolated from ear in most cases
   (iii) Presents as bacterial otitis externa with granulations in
        canal
   (iv) Progresses to fulminating perichondritis of pinna and
        necrotising osteitis of skull base
   (v) Complications include lateral sinus thrombosis, petrous
        apicitis, meningitis, cerebral abscess and carotis artery
        rupture
   (vi) Cranial nerve palsies common in advanced stages, e.g. VII
        nerve, jugular fossa syndrome

With multiple cranial nerve palsies the mortality rate is 80%

2. Treatment
   (i) Early disease
        a. Hospitalisation
        b. Repeated aural toilet and removal of granulatioms
        c. Topical gentamicin and parenteral gentamicin and
           carbenicillin
   (ii) Advanced disease (or if no response after 72 hours of
        antibiotics)
        a. Wide excision of infected cartilage, soft tissue and bone
        b. Mastoidectomy if radiological evidence of mastoiditis
   (iii) Antibiotic treatment should continue for at least 1 month

3. **Differential diagnosis of bleeding granulations in the external auditory canal**
    (i) Bacterial otitis externa
    (ii) Malignant otitis externa
    (iii) Granulomatous disease, e.g. tuberculosis, Wegener's granuloma
    (iv) Squamous cell carcinoma
    (v) Glomus tumour

BAROTRAUMA

A sudden increase in atmospheric pressure may have a variety of effects on the ear

1. Secretory otitis media (with or without haemotympanum)
2. TM perforation
3. Ossicular disruption
4. Labyrinthine membrane rupture
5. Sensorineural hearing loss
6. Vestibular dysfunction

BULLOUS MYRINGITIS

Clinical features
    (i) Often associated with influenza epidemic
    (ii) Children and young adults affected
    (iii) Severe otalgia associated with haemorrhagic bullae on the tympanic membrane
    (iv) Serosanguineous otorrhoea occurs when bullae burst
    (v) Deafness only occurs if a middle ear effusion develops (10%)
    (vi) Secondary bacterial infection of bullae can occur

Otorrhoea

DISCHARGE FROM THE EAR

The discharge may consist of pus, blood, serous fluid, perilymph or cerebrospinal fluid

CAUSES

1. Infective
    (i) Otitis externa
    (ii) Myringitis
    (iii) Acute suppurative otitis media
    (iv) Chronic suppurative otitis media
    (v) Infected mastoid or fenestration cavity

2. Traumatic
    (i) Foreign body
    (ii) Head injury
    (iii) Instrumentation
    (iv) Barotrauma
    (v) Temporal bone fracture

3. Neoplastic
    Squamous cell carcinoma of middle ear

INVESTIGATIONS

1. History
    (i) Onset
    (ii) Duration
    (iii) Otalgia
    (iv) Hearing loss
    (v) Vertigo
    (vi) Trauma
    (vii) Recent upper respiratory tract infection
    (viii) Otitis media in childhood
    (ix) Previous aural surgery

2. Examination
- (i) Ears
- (ii) Nose
- (iii) Oral cavity and oropharynx
- (iv) Cranial nerves

3. Investigations
- (i) Haematology
  - a. FBC + ESR
  - b. Blood sugar
- (ii) Radiology
  - a. Mastoid X-rays
  - b. Mastoid tomography
  - c. Skull X-rays
  - d. Sinus X-rays
  - e. CT Scan of head
- (iii) Bacteriology — Aural swab
  - a. Aerobes
  - b. Anaerobes
  - c. Fungi and yeasts
- (iv) Audiology
  - a. PTA
  - b. Tympanometry
- (v) Surgical
  - a. Suction clearance
  - b. Biopsy

The choice of investigations is determined by the clinical findings

ACUTE SUPPURATIVE OTITIS MEDIA

1. Causes
- (i) Common cold
- (ii) Acute or chronic sinusitis
- (iii) Acute or chronic tonsillitis or nasopharyngitis
- (iv) Influenza, measles or chicken pox

2. Stages
- (i) Tubal occlusion: acute salpingitis
- (ii) Presuppuration: hyperaemia of middle ear mucosa with middle ear exudate
- (iii) Suppuration: bulging and perforation of tympanic membrane
- (iv) Resolution: under favourable conditions the tympanic membrane perforation heals

3. **Clinical features**
    (i)   Otalgia (prior to suppuration)
    (ii) Pyrexia
    (iii) Red bulging tympanic membrane
    (iv) Conductive hearing loss
    (v)   Otorrhoea (marks onset of suppurative stage)
    (vi) Causative organism
        a. B haemolytic streptococci
        b. *Strep. pneumoniae*
        c. *Staph. albus* and *Staph. aureus*
        d. *Haemophilus influenzae*

4. **Causes of recurrent acute suppurative otitis media**
    (i)   Chronic Eustachian tube dysfunction
    (ii) Persistant fluid in the middle ear cleft
    (iii) Persistant focus of infection in the upper respiratory tract
    (iv) Mastoid reservoir

5. **Sequelae of acute suppurative otitis media**
    (i)   Healing of tympanic membrane with normal hearing
    (ii)   Glue ear
    (iii) Chronic suppurative otitis media
    (iv)   Adhesive otitis media
    (v)   Tympanosclerosis
    (vi)   Ossicular destruction
    (vii) Acute mastoiditis
    (viii) Intratemporal or intracranial complications

CHRONIC SUPPURATIVE OTITIS MEDIA

Table 6 Clinical features

	Safe (Tubo-tympanic)	Unsafe (Attico-antral)
Aetiology	Recurrent acute suppurative otitis media Exanthemata	Eustachian tube dysfunction with formation of an attic retraction pocket or perforation Abnormal epithelial migration
Otalgia	Mild	Moderate
Otorrhoea	Profuse mucopurulent	Scanty and offensive *Pseudomonas/Proteus*
Typical appearance of tympanic membrane	Central perforation	Marginal perforation with cholesteatoma and aural polyp

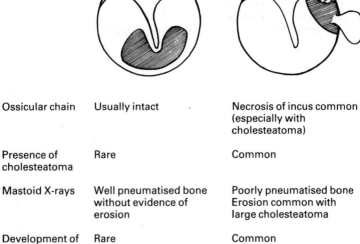

Ossicular chain	Usually intact	Necrosis of incus common (especially with cholesteatoma)
Presence of cholesteatoma	Rare	Common
Mastoid X-rays	Well pneumatised bone without evidence of erosion	Poorly pneumatised bone Erosion common with large cholesteatoma
Development of intratemporal or intracranial complications	Rare	Common

1. **Clinical staging of chronic suppurative otitis media**
    (i) Active state — The ear is discharging pus
    (ii) Quiescent state — The ear is not discharging but has recently been doing so and has a history or recurrent discharge
    (iii) Inactive state — There is a past history of discharge but the ear is now dry and has been for a significant period of time
    (iv) Healed state — The ear is permanently dry, the perforation having healed or been repaired

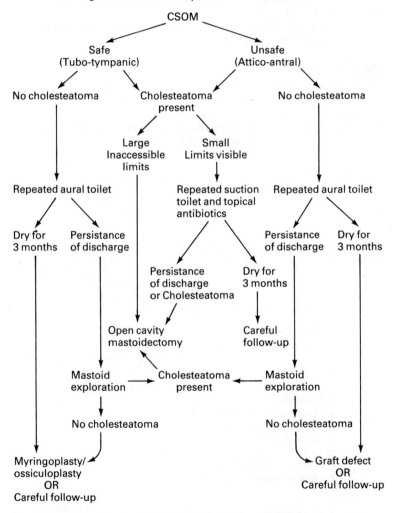

Fig. 10 Treatment of chronic suppurative otitis media (CSOM)

IN CHILDREN 25% OF ALL BRAIN ABSCESSES ARE OTOGENIC
AND IN ADULTS 50% ARE OTOGENIC. THEY CAN BE
CEREBELLAR OR TEMPORAL LOBE IN SITE AND CARRY A
MORTALITY RATE OF 40%

2. **Complications of acute and chronic suppurative otitis media and mastoiditis**

   (i) *Intratemporal*
       a. Facial palsy
       b. Labyrinthitis (spread of infection commonly via lateral semicircular canal)

Table 7 Labyrinthitis

	Pathology	Clinical features
Paralabyrinthitis	Mucoperiosteum of canal exposed, but no cells in perilymph	Fistula sign positive
Serous labyrinthitis	Serous exudate present in perilymph	Spontaneous nausea and vomiting with irritative nystagmus to infected side Reversible
Suppurative labyrinthitis	Suppuration within labyrinth	Symptoms of acute vestibular failure with paralytic nystagmus away from infected side Irreversible

       c. Petrositis
       d. Gradenigo's syndrome — Otorrhoea
                                  Ipsilateral VIth nerve palsy
                                  Pain in the distribution of the
                                  ipsilateral Vth nerve
   (ii) *Intracranial*
       a. Extradural abscess
       b. Subdural abscess
       c. Meningitis
       d. Venous sinus thrombosis
       e. Otitic hydrocephalus
       f. Brain abscess

CHOLESTEATOMA

When stratified squamous epithelium in the middle ear cleft forms a matrix which continually desquamates concentric sheets of keratin into a confined space or pocket a cholesteatoma develops

Theories of cholesteatoma development
  (i) The immigration theory
     a. Direct ingrowth of squamous epithelium through a perforation
     b. Proliferation and ingrowth of a solid core of squamous epithelium into the attic region
     c. Development within a pre-existing skin lined retraction pocket
 (ii) The metaplasia theory
(iii) The implantation theory
(iv) The congenital theory

ACQUIRED CHOLESTEATOMA IS COMMONLY FOUND IN ASSOCIATION WITH UNSAFE CSOM. HOWEVER, IT IS OCCASIONALLY FOUND IN CASES OF SAFE CSOM

TUBERCULOUS OTITIS MEDIA

Clinical features
  (i) Most common in children
 (ii) Spread usually from chest via nasopharynx
(iii) Chronic insidious course most common
(iv) Otorrhoea but characteristically no otalgia
 (v) Severe deafness
(vi) Multiple tympanic membrane perforations coalescing to form a large single perforation
(vii) Cervical lymphadenopathy
(viii) Complications such as facial palsy, meningitis or labyrinthitis often develop without preceding symptoms

TYMPANOSCLEROSIS

This is an irreversible, benign condition which is one of the possible results of the middle ears response to repeated inflammation. The inflammatory infiltrate in the middle ear cleft mucosa becomes invaded by fibroblasts with the development of areas of collagenous connective tissue which undergo hyalin degeneration and calcification

THE TYMPANIC MEMBRANE REMAINS INTACT IN 40% OF CASES

Causes of resultant conductive hearing loss
  (i) Malleus head fixation
  (ii) Stapes ankylosis
  (iii) Ossicular destruction
  (iv) Tympanic membrane immobility
  (v) Round window occlusion

CSF OTORRHOEA

Causes
  (i) Temporal bone fracture
  (ii) Iatrogenic
  (iii) Cholesteatoma
  (iv) Tumour
  (v) Congenital defect

Table 8 Temporal bone fractures

	Incidence (%)	Associated with facial palsy (%)	Other features
Longitudinal	80	20	Torn tympanic membrane Bleeding from ear Conductive hearing loss
Transverse	20	50	Intact tympanic membrane Haemotympanum Sensorineural hearing loss and vertigo

A CSF LEAK FROM A DEFECT IN THE TEMPORAL BONE MAY PRESENT AS CSF RHINORRHOEA

Vertigo

AN HALLUCINATION OF MOVEMENT

The movement need not be rotatory

CAUSES

1. Central
- (i) Traumatic — Head injury
- (ii) Infective
  - a. Meningitis
  - b. Brain abscess
- (iii) Neoplastic
  - a. Glioma
  - b. Cerebral secondary
- (iv) Vascular — Vertebrobasilar insufficiency
- (v) Miscellaneous
  - a. Multiple sclerosis
  - b. Epilepsy

2. Peripheral
- (i) Traumatic
  - a. Head injury
  - b. Barotrauma
  - c. Labyrinthine membrane rupture
  - d. Iatrogenic
- (ii) Infective
  - a. Bacterial labyrinthitis
  - b. Viral labyrinthitis
  - c. Syphilis
  - d. Vestibular neuronitis
  - e. *Herpes zoster oticus*
  - f. Suppurative otitis media
- (iii) Neoplastic
  - a. Benign — Acoustic neuroma
  - b. Malignant — SCCa middle ear
- (iv) Metabolic — Menière's disease
- (v) Toxins — Vestibulotoxic drugs

(vi) Miscellaneous
   a. Benign positional vertigo
   b. Otosclerosis

> OVER 80% OF THE PATIENTS WHO PRESENT WITH VERTIGO
> HAVE A PERIPHERAL CAUSE

INVESTIGATION

1. History
   (i) Onset
   (ii) Duration
   (iii) Periodicity
   (iv) Hearing loss
   (v) Tinnitus
   (vi) Otorrhoea
   (vii) Loss of consciousness
   (viii) Other neurological symptoms
   (ix) Ototoxic drugs
   (x) Head injury

2. Examination
   (i) Ears
   (ii) Neurological
   (iii) Neck: bruits
   (iv) Positional tests

3. Investigations
   (i) Haematology
      a. FBC + ESR
      b. VDRL / TPHA
   (ii) Radiology
      a. Mastoid X-rays
      b. Internal auditory meatus X-rays
      c. CT scan
   (iii) Audiology
      a. PTA
      b. Speech audiometry
      c. Loudness balance
      d. Reflex decay
      e. Evoked response audiometry
   (iv) Vestibular function studies:
      a. Electromystagmography at rest and on caloric testing
      b. Positional testing
   (v) Others — Glycerol dehydration test

The choice of investigations is determined by the clinical findings

Eye closure enhances peripheral vertigo whilst optic fixation enhances central vertigo

Maintainance of balance and posture at rest or during movement requires intact visual, proprioceptive and vestibular systems. If a fault occurs in any one of these systems normal equilibrium is disrupted and imbalance results. Nystagmus can occur if there is disruption of the ocular, vestibular or cerebellar pathways

At rest both vestibular labyrinths maintain a constant baseline neural discharge. Acceleration of the body in one direction increases the neural discharge from one or more of the cristae on one side, whilst proportionately decreasing the output from the cristae on the other side. The resulting imbalance in the stimulation of the two groups of vestibular nuclei and their higher centres results in vertigo. This vertigo persists for the duration of the stimulus (it will cease if a constant speed is attained but will recur if further acceleration or decelleration follows)

When unilateral acute vestibular failure occurs (eg. following surgical labyrinthectomy) then the resulting vertigo will persist for 4–6 weeks whilst three compensating mechanisms help to restore equilibrium and balance
   (i) Temporary 'cerebellar clampdown' on the normally discharging contralateral vestibular nuclei
  (ii) Generation of a new resting neural activity in the non-functioning ipsilateral vestibular nuclei
 (iii) Reprogramming of central centres to readapt to the new neural inputs

If the output of one labyrinth is constantly changing (e.g. following an incomplete surgical labyrinthectomy) then full compensation cannot be achieved and the patient will suffer from chronic vertigo

THE FITZGERALD-HALLPIKE CALORIC TEST
A comparison of the durations of nystagmus obtained by warm water (44°C) and cold water (30°C) stimulation of the endolymph in each of the lateral semicircular canals provides an assessment of function of both vestibular labyrinths and their central connections (Fig. 11)

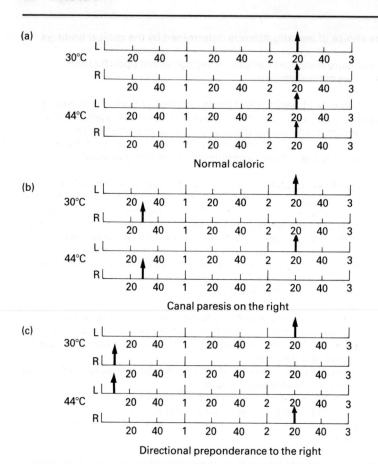

Fig. 11 (a) A normal caloric. (b) A canal paresis on the right exists when cold and warm water stimulation of the right ear produce the same reduction in the duration of nystagmus. It indicates a peripheral vestibular lesion. (c) A directional preponderance to the right exists when the duration of nystagmus produced by warm water in the right ear and cold water in the left is greater than the duration of the nystagmus produced by cold water in the right ear and warm water in the left. A directional preponderance can be the result of a central or a peripheral vestibular lesion

Nystagmus
  (i) Physiological
  (ii) Pathological
    a. Ocular
    b. Vestibular
    c. Cerebellar

Spontaneous vestibular nystagmus can be
a. 1° — only occurs when eyes deviated in the direction of the fast component
b. 2° — occurs on looking straight ahead as well
c. 3° — also seen when eyes deviated in direction of slow component

LABYRINTHINE MEMBRANE RUPTURE

The perilymph leak usually occurs through the round window

1. **Mechanism**
   (i) Explosive — Due to a sudden rise in cerebrospinal fluid pressure in relation to middle ear pressure, e.g. head injury, barotrauma, physical exertion
   (ii) Implosive — Due to a sudden rise in middle ear pressure in relation to cerebrospinal fluid pressure, e.g. direct blow to ear, forced Valsalvas manoeuvre

2. **Clinical features**
   (i) Sudden onset deafness which may fluctuate
   (ii) Vertigo, which can be positional, intermittant or chronic
   (iii) Evidence of fluid in the middle ear may be present
   (iv) Fistula test may be positive
   (v) PTA shows a sensorineural or mixed hearing loss

MENIÈRE'S DISEASE

After presbyacusis and noise induced hearing loss Menière's disease is the most common disorder of the inner ear. It is the most common cause of peripheral vertigo

1. **Clinical varieties**
   (i) Classical Menière's disease
      a. Paroxysms of vertigo in association with hearing loss
      b. The vertigo may overshadow the other features of tinnitus and 'fullness' in the ear
   (ii) Lermoyez syndrome — The hearing improves during and immediately after the attack of vertigo
   (iii) Vestibular Menière's disease — Hearing loss is not a feature
   (iv) Cochlear Menière's disease — Paroxysmal vertigo is not a feature

2. **Clinical Features**
   (i) Affects approximately 0.1% of the population
   (ii) Very rare in children
   (iii) 80% of cases initially unilateral
   (iv) Affects both sexes equally

   (v) Attacks often occur in clusters with prolonged periods of
       remission in between
  (vi) During periods of remission the hearing loss may continue
       to fluctuate
 (vii) Audiologically the deafness is cochlear in type
(viii) Electrocochleography shows characteristic changes.
  (ix) A positive glycerol dehydration test occurs in about 60% of
       patients in the early stages and is diagnostic of Menières
       disease
   (x) In longstanding cases the vertigo becomes less severe but
       the hearing loss and tinnitus become progressively worse

3. Treatment
   (i) Medical
      a. Labyrinthine sedatives
      b. Salt restriction with or without a diuretic
      c. Vasodilators

Table 9 Comparison of Menière's disease and acoustic neuroma

	Menière's disease	Acoustic neuroma
Site of lesion	Cochlea Eventually bilateral in 50%	Retrocochlear Rarely bilateral
Pathophysiology	Paroxysmal distension of the membranous labyrinth	Benign Schwann cell tumour
Clinical features	Episodic vertigo, hearing loss, tinnitus and fullness in the ear. Attacks occur in clusters and last 2–12 hours	Otological phase followed by neurological phase
Audiometry PTA	Initially a low frequency sensorineural hearing loss	Initially a high frequency sensorineural hearing loss
Other	Recruiting deafness	Non-recruiting deafness Adaptation tests +ve
ERA	Characteristic ECoG	Characteristic BSER
Fitzgerald-Hallpike Caloric	Abnormal in 50%	Abnormal in 95%
Temporal bone radiology	Normal	IAM tomography and CT scanning usually abnormal

(ii) Surgical
    a. Conservative — Grommet insertion
                  — Saccus decompression
    b. Destructive — Vestibular nerve section
                 — Labyrinthectomy

ACUTE VESTIBULAR FAILURE

1. With normal cochlear function — Idiopathic acute vestibular failure (acute viral labyrinthitis)
   Clinical features
   (i) Sudden onset of severe vertigo
   (ii) Often associated with an upper respiratory tract infection
   (iii) Vertigo settles over 7–10 days but imbalance lasts 3–4 weeks
   (iv) Caloric test shows a partial or complete canal paresis which does not recover
2. With associated sudden sensorineural hearing loss
   (i) Temporal bone fracture
   (ii) Suppurative labyrinthitis
   (iii) Vascular occlusion
   (iv) Iatrogenic
   (v) Idiopathic

OTOTOXIC DRUGS

1. Aminoglycoside antibiotics — Damage the neuroepithelial hair cells in the crista ampullaris, macula and Organ of Corti. The stria vascularis may also be affected. Toxic effects are more likely to occur in patients with impaired renal function
   (i) Streptomycin
   (ii) Gentamicin   Primarily vestibulotoxic
   (iii) Kanamycin
   (iv) Neomycin   Primarily cochleotoxic

   The vestibular dysfunction or deafness are rarely reversible. Symptoms can commence or persist several months after finishing treatment

2. Diuretics
   (i) Both ethacrynic acid and frusemide can cause deafness by damaging the stria vascularis
   (ii) The deafness is often reversible in the early stages
3. Salicylates — Very high doses can cause deafness and tinnitus which are usually reversible
4. Quinine — Can cause deafness, which is usually reversible.

BENIGN POSITIONAL VERTIGO

Recurrent, transient episodes of vertigo which only occur when the head assumes certain positions

1. **Causes**
     (i) Idiopathic
    (ii) Head Injury
   (iii) Suppurative ear disease
   (iv) Post stapedectomy

2. **Clinical features**
     (i) Characteristic history of vertigo in certain head positions, often occurring in bed
    (ii) Can often be precipitated by positional testing, with symptoms and nystagmus following a latent period
   (iii) Transient nystagmus abating after 30–40 seconds
   (iv) Response fatigues after repeated testing
    (v) Associated with violent vertigo, nausea and vomiting

Tinnitus

THE SUBJECTIVE EXPERIENCE OF HEARING SIMPLE SOUNDS IN THE EAR OR HEAD

Subjective tinnitus can rarely also be objective

CAUSES

1. **Central**
   - (i) Cerebrovascular disease
   - (ii) Tumour

2. **Retrocochlear**
   - (i) Cerebello-pontine angle tumour e.g. acoustic neuroma
   - (ii) Syphilis

3. **Cochlear**
   - (i) Idiopathic
   - (ii) Menière's disease
   - (iii) Presbyacusis
   - (iv) Noise induced hearing loss
   - (v) Ototoxic drugs
   - (vi) High cardiac output states

4. **Conductive**
   - (i) Wax
   - (ii) Middle ear effusion e.g. acute otitis media, glue ear
   - (iii) Chronic suppurative otitis media
   - (iv) Otosclerosis
   - (v) Iatrogenic e.g. following myringoplasty, stapedectomy, insertion of grommet
   - (vi) Glomus tumour
   - (vii) Palatal myoclonus
   - (viii) Costens syndrome
   - (ix) Vascular anomalies in the occipito-mastoid region

Tinnitus can accompany most otological diseases. The importance attached to the symptom varies with the individual patient

INVESTIGATIONS

A distinction must be made between tinnitus, where the sound is simple, and auditory hallucination where the patient experiences far more complex sounds such as speech. Auditory hallucination is a psychiatric phenomenon

1. History
  (i) Onset
  (ii) Duration
  (iii) Description of tinnitus
  (iv) Progression
  (v) Relation to stress
  (vi) Hearing loss or vertigo
  (vii) Noise exposure
  (viii) Drugs

2. Examination
  (i) Ears
  (ii) Nose
  (iii) Neurological
  (iv) Neck (bruits)

3. Investigations
  (i) Haematology
    a. FBC + ESR
    b. VDRL/TPHA
  (ii) Radiology
    a. Skull base X-rays
    b. Mastoid X-rays
    c. IAM X-rays
  (iii) Audiology
    a. PTA
    b. Tympanometry
  (iv) Other — Caloric tests

The choice of investigations is determined by the clinical findings

> IT IS ESSENTIAL TO EXCLUDE ANY ORGANIC DISEASE ALTHOUGH MOST CASES OF TINNITUS ARE IDIOPATHIC

GLOMUS TUMOUR

Clinical features
1. A slow growing tumour of paraganglionic tissue which rarely metastasizes
2. More common in women (75%)
3. Associated with chemodectomas elsewhere
4. Commonly occur in jugular bulb (glomus jugulare) or on the promontory (glomus tympanicum)
5. Symptoms
     (i) Aural
     (ii) Cranial nerve palsies
     (iii) Intracranial
6. Radiologically diagnosed by jugular fossa tomography and arteriography

Facial palsy

The cause may be upper or lower motor neurone disease

CAUSES

1. **Congenital**
   Birth trauma

2. **Acquired**
   (i) Intracranial
      a. Neoplastic — Acoustic neuroma
                      Meningioma
      b. Infective — Meningitis
      c. Traumatic — Neurosurgical
      d. Miscellaneous — Cerebrovascular occlusion
                         Multiple sclerosis
   (ii) Intratemporal
      a. Traumatic — Mastoid surgery
                     Temporal bone fracture
      b. Infective — Acute otitis media
                     Chronic otitis media with cholesteatoma
                     Herpes zoster oticus
      c. Neoplastic — Benign — Facial nerve neuroma
                      Malignant — Squamous cell carcinoma
      d. Miscellaneous — Bell's palsy
   (iii) Peripheral
      a. Traumatic — Parotid gland surgery
                     Facial laceration
      b. Neoplastic — Parotid gland malignancy

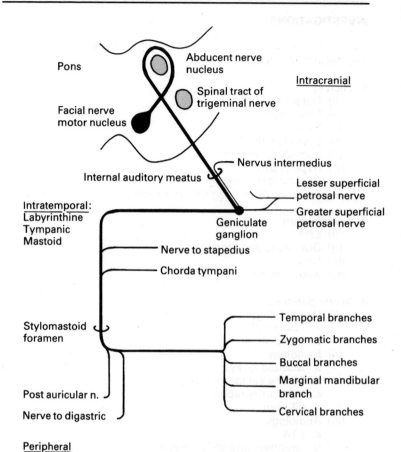

Fig. 12 Anatomy of the facial nerve

INVESTIGATIONS

95% OF FACIAL NERVE PALSIES ARE DUE TO A LESION WITHIN
THE TEMPORAL BONE

1. History
    (i) Duration
    (ii) Progression
    (iii) Pain
    (iv) Loss of taste
    (v) Loss of lacrimation
    (vi) Hyperacusis
    (vii) Hearing loss or vertigo
    (viii) Associated neurological symptoms

2. Examination
    (i) Ears
    (ii) Oral cavity and oropharynx
    (iii) Neck
    (iv) Neurological

3. Investigations
    (i) Haematology
        a. FBC + ESR
        b. Blood sugar
    (ii) Radiology
        a. Mastoid X-rays
        b. Middle ear tomography
        c. IAM tomography
        d. CT scan
    (iii) Audiology
        a. PTA
        b. Loudness discomfort levels
        c. Acoustic reflexes
    (iv) Others
        a. Schirmer's test
        b. Electrogustometry
        c. Submandibular gland duct salivary flow rates
        d. Electrophysiological studies

> IMMEDIATE POST-OPERATIVE FACIAL PALSY FOLLOWING
> MIDDLE EAR SURGERY REQUIRES IMMEDIATE RE-EXPLORATION
> OF THE EAR

The choice of investigations is determined by the clinical findings

ELECTROPHYSIOLOGICAL ASSESSMENT OF FACIAL NERVE FUNCTION

1. *Nerve excitability test*
   Three days after the onset of the palsy, the stimulation thresholds of both facial nerves are measured. If the threshold on the side of the palsy is raised by more than 4–5 mA then the nerve function is significantly impaired

2. *Electromyography*
   Normal facial nerve function is characterised by insertion potentials and motor unit potentials recorded during facial movement. Approximately 15–20 days following nerve degeneration, spontaneous fibrillation potentials develop. These eventually cease in the longstanding facial palsy. Polyphasic motor unit potentials indicate reinnervation and preceed obvious return of facial movement

3. *Electroneuronography*
   Supramaximal stimulation of the nerve at the stylomastoid foramen produces a muscle action potential recorded in the nasolabial fold. By comparing the height of the action potential on the abnormal side with the height of the potential on the normal side the percentage loss of nerve fibres can be estimated as early as 48 hours after onset of the palsy. If less than 5% of the nerve fibres are surviving at 2 weeks then the prognosis for good recovery of function is very poor

---

BELL'S PALSY IS THE MOST COMMON CAUSE OF FACIAL PARALYSIS

Table 10 Comparison of Bell's palsy and *Herpes zoster oticus*

	Bell's palsy (Idiopathic facial palsy)	***Herpes zoster oticus*** (Ramsay Hunt syndrome)
Predisposing factors	Pregnancy Diabetes mellitus	Underlying malignant disease
Site of involvement	Usually below geniculate ganglion	Geniculate ganglion
Other cranial nerve palsies	No	VIII most frequent IX and X nerve palsies may occur V, VI and XII nerve palsies are more rare
Prodromal illness	No	Preceeding fever and malaise common
Pain	Uncommon (but associated with poor prognosis)	Very common (may proceed facial palsy by 2–4 days)
Hearing loss/ vertigo	No	Common
Loss of taste	In half of the cases	Very common
Loss of lacrimation	Uncommon	Common
Chance of complete recovery (%)	90	60
Treatment	The treatment is the same for both conditions	

No treatment is required for a partial nerve palsy as full recovery can always be expected. The role of corticosteroids for the complete palsy remains unsettled, as does the place of surgical decompression of the nerve. Some otologists recommend surgical decompression at 2 weeks if electroneuronography demonstrates less than 5% functioning nerve fibres

PART TWO

The nose and paranasal sinuses

Anatomy

BONES CONSTITUTING THE LATERAL WALL OF THE NOSE

1. Maxilla
2. Perpendicular plate of palatine bone
3. Nasal surface of lacrimal bone
4. Ethmoid bone
     (i) Uncinate process
     (ii) Middle and superior turbinate
     (iii) Bulla
5. Inferior turbinates
6. Medial pterygoid plate
7. Nasal bone

CONSTITUENTS OF THE NASAL SEPTUM

1. Bones
     (i) Perpendicular plate of ethmoid
     (ii) Vomer
2. Quadrilateral cartilage

STRUCTURE OPENING INTO THE SPHENOETHMOIDAL RECESS

Sphenoid sinus

STRUCTURES OPENING INTO THE SUPERIOR MEATUS

1. Posterior ethmoidal cells
2. Sphenopalatine foramen

STRUCTURES OPENING INTO THE MIDDLE MEATUS

1. Frontal sinus
2. Anterior ethmoidal cells
3. Maxillary sinus
4. Middle ethmoidal cells

STRUCTURE OPENING INTO THE INFERIOR MEATUS

1. Nasolacrimal duct

Table 11 Arteries supplying the nose

Anterior	Posterior
Lateral wall	
Ant ethmoidal	Post sup lat nasal aa
Ant Sup alveolar	Brs of greater palatine
Septum	
Ant ethmoidal	Long sphenopalatine
Septal br of superior labial	Ascending branches of greater palatine

Table 12 Nerves supplying the nose

Anterior	Posterior
Lateral wall	
Ant ethmoidal	Lat nasal branches of sphenopalatine
Ant sup alveolar	Branches of greater palatine
Septum	
Ant ethmoidal	Nasopalatine

LYMPHATIC DRAINAGE OF THE NASAL CAVITIES

1. Anterior — To submandibular nodes in vessels accompanying anterior facial veins
2. Posterior — To retropharyngeal and upper deep cervical nodes

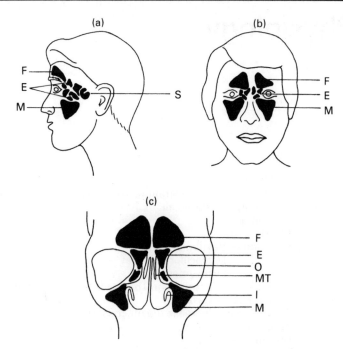

Fig. 13 The paranasal sinuses. F = frontal sinus; E = ethmoid air cells; S = spheroid sinus; M = maxillary antrum; O = orbit; MT = middle turbinate; I = inferior turbinate (c) coronal section showing relationship of paranasal sinuses to the orbit

Physiology

1. **Functions of the nose**
   - (i) Respiration — Nasal respiration is obligate in the newborn
   - (ii) Conditioning of inspired air
     - a. Warming
     - b. Moistening
     - c. Filtration — Vestibular hairs
       Mucociliary blanket
       Lysozymes
     - d. Nasal airflow is turbulent. This leads to greater contact with mucosal surfaces
     - e. The turbinates increase the mucosal surface area
     - f. When inspired air reaches the pharynx —
       Humidity is > 75%
       Temperature = 36°C
       Most particulate matter has been removed
   - (iii) Olfaction (Smell)
     - a. In quiet respiration 5–10% of the inspired air passes through the olfactory cleft
     - b. During sniffing up to 20% of the inspired air passes through the olfactory cleft

2. **Disturbances of smell**
   - (i) Hyposmia — Partial quantitative loss of smell
     Causes
     - a. Nasal obstruction
     - b. Olfactory nerve trauma
     - c. Olfactory tract compression by tumour
   - (ii) Anosmia — Complete absence of smell
     Causes
     - a. Congenital
     - b. Acquired — Olfactory nerve shearing by head injury
       Olfactory nerve/tract damaged by tumour

(iii) Cacosmia — Unpleasant smell due to noxious substance in
nose
Causes
a. Maxillary sinusitis
b. Foreign body in the nose
c. Chronic middle ear infection
(iv) Parosmia — Sensation of unpleasant smell in absence of
noxious substance within nose
Causes
a. Functional
b. Organic — Temporal lobe epilepsy
Streptomycin

Radiology

1. **Conventional radiology**
    (i) Occipito-mental view — (Water's)
        a. Maxillary antra
        b. Frontal sinus
        c. Sphenoid sinus
    (ii) Lateral view
        a. Sphenoid sinus
        b. Frontal sinus
        c. Ethmoid sinus
        d. Post-nasal space
        e. Nasal bones
    (iii) Submento-vertical view
        a. Sphenoid sinus
        b. Ethmoid sinus
        c. Maxillary antra
    (iv) Occipito-frontal view — (Caldwell)
        a. Frontal sinus
        b. Ethmoid sinus
        c. Nasal cavity
        d. Orbital margins

2. **Tomography**
    (i) Fractures
    (ii) Bony destruction
    (iii) Tumours

3. **CT Scan —**
    Tumours

4. **Carotid arteriography**
    (i) Nasopharyngeal angiofibroma
    (ii) Epistaxis

Nasal obstruction

CONGENITAL

1. Posterior choanal atresia
2. Nasal glioma

ACQUIRED

1. Acute
  (i) Infective
    a. Viral
    b. Bacterial
  (ii) Traumatic
    a. Foreign body
    b. Septal haematoma
    c. Septal deviation

2. Chronic
  (i) Structural — Septal deviation
  (ii) Polyposis
    a. Nasal
    b. Antrochoanal
  (iii) Rhinitis
    a. Infective
    b. Vasomotor
    c. Allergic
    d. Atrophic
  (iv) 2° infection
    a. Sinusitis
    b. Adenoids
  (v) Neoplastic
    a. Nose — Papilloma
            Inverted papilloma
            Squamous carcinoma

b. PNS — Juvenile angiofibroma
   Squamous carcinoma
   Lymphoma
c. Sinuses — Squamous carcinoma
(vi) Granulomatous
   a. TB
   b. Sarcoid
   c. Wegener's
(vii) Iatrogenic — Rhinitis medicamentosa
(viii) Foreign Body — Rhinolith

COMMON CAUSES OF NASAL OBSTRUCTION

1. Unilateral
   (i) Deviated nasal septum
   (ii) Foreign body
   (iii) Tumour of nasal cavity or paranasal sinus

2. Bilateral
   (i) Child — Adenoidal hypertrophy
   (ii) Adult
      a. Nasal polyps
      b. Vasomotor/allergic rhinitis

UNILATERAL BLOODY NASAL DISCHARGE

1. Child — Foreign body
2. Adult — Tumour of nose or sinuses

FOREIGN BODY IN THE NOSE

1. Children
   (i) Organic vegetable matter — Unilateral purulent discharge
   (ii) Inert — May be asymptomatic

2. Adults — Rhinolith — Calcareous mass presenting as chronic
                           unilateral foul-smelling bloodstained
                           nasal discharge

FOREIGN BODIES IN THE NOSE SHOULD ALWAYS BE REMOVED
TO PREVENT DISLODGEMENT AND INHALATION

CHOANAL ATRESIA

Absent canalisation of the posterior choanae of the nose resulting
from failure of the buccopharyngeal membrane to rupture in
embryonic life

1. **General features**
    (i) May be unilateral or bilateral (65% are unilateral)
    (ii) May be complete or incomplete
    (iii) May be bony or membranous (90% are bony)
    (iv) Incidence 1:60,000 live births
    (v) Occurs twice as commonly in females
    (vi) 50% have other associated congenital abnormalities

2. **Presentation**
    (i) Unilateral — Chronic nasal discharge in childhood
    (ii) Bilateral — Airway emergency in the newborn
            Extreme feeding difficulties

NASAL BREATHING IS OBLIGATE IN THE NEWBORN

3. **Diagnosis**
    (i) Passage of a fine rubber catheter
    (ii) Instillation of radio-opaque dye

4. **Management**
    (i) Unilateral — Surgical correction from one year onwards
    (ii) Bilateral
        a. Initial — Oral airway
        b. Definitive — Surgical correction — Transnasal approach
                                                                Transpalatal
                                                                approach

NB after surgical correction intranasal silastic tubing maintains nasal
patency for the first 3 months

NASAL POLYPS

1. **Simple ethmoidal polyps**
    Pedunculated oedematous swellings of the mucosal lining of the
    ethmoidal cells that cascade into the nose from below the middle
    turbinate
    (i) General features
        a. Pearly and smooth
        b. Often multiple
        c. Usually bilateral
        d. Recurrent
    (ii) Contributing factors
        a. Allergic rhinitis
        b. Chronic sinusitis

NASAL POLYPOSIS IN CHILDREN MAY BE ASSOCIATED WITH CYSTIC FIBROSIS

(iii) Symptoms
    a. Nasal obstruction
    b. Loss of smell
    c. Postnasal drip
    d. Clear rhinorrhoea
    e. Sneezing

(iv) Treatment

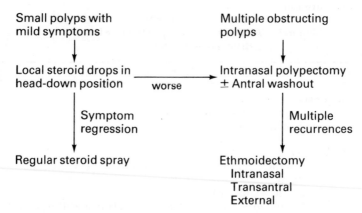

Small polyps with mild symptoms	Multiple obstructing polyps
↓	↓
Local steroid drops in head-down position ——worse——→	Intranasal polypectomy ± Antral washout
↓ Symptom regression	↓ Multiple recurrences
Regular steroid spray	Ethmoidectomy Intranasal Transantral External

2. Antrochoanal polyps
Mucosal polyps which originate from the maxillary antrum and extend through the maxillary ostium to pass through the posterior choana and enter the nasopharynx
  (i) General features
    a. Occur in the 10–30 age group
    b. Usually unilateral
    c. Aetiology unclear
  (ii) Symptoms
    a. Unilateral nasal obstruction initially
    b. Postnasal drip
    c. Nasal voice
    d. Bilateral nasal obstruction later
    e. Lump in the throat when very large
  (iii) Treatment — Surgical removal
    a. Avulsion
    b. Caldwell Luc approach for recurrences

3. Neoplastic polyps
Some tumours have a polypoid appearance and therefore occasionally may be confused with simple nasal polyps

  (i) Benign
 a. Inverted papilloma
 b. Neurofibroma
 c. Meningioma
 d. Olfactory neuroblastoma
 e. Nasal glioma (children)
 (ii) Malignant
 a. Carcinoma
 b. Melanoma

UNILATERAL SWELLINGS IN THE NOSE SHOULD ALWAYS BE BIOPSIED

TUMOURS OF THE NOSE AND PARANASAL SINUSES

Less than 1% of all tumours

1. Benign
  (i) Epithelial
 a. Adenoma
 b. Squamous papilloma
 c. Inverted papilloma — (Ringert's tumour)
 (ii) Mesenchymal
 a. Osteoma
 b. Chondroma

2. Malignant
  (i) Epithelial
 a. Squamous cell carcinoma
 b. Anaplastic carcinoma
 c. Transitional cell carcinoma
 d. Primary adenocarcinoma
 e. Secondary adenocarcinoma — Renal
              Gastrointestinal tract
 (ii) Lymphoid — Reticuloses
(iii) Mesenchymal
 a. Osteosarcoma
 b. Chondrosarcoma
 c. Fibrosarcoma
(iv) Salivary tumours
 a. Adenoid cystic carcinoma
 b. Mucoepidermoid carcinoma
 (v) Neural crest
 a. Melanoma
 b. Olfactory neuroblastoma

80% OF PARANASAL SINUS TUMOURS ARE SQUAMOUS CELL CARCINOMA

SYMPTOMS OF PARANASAL SINUS AND NASAL TUMOURS

1. Nose (44%)
    (i) Nasal obstruction
    (ii) Purulent nasal secretion
    (iii) Bloody nasal secretion

2. Face (33%)
    (i) Facial pain
    (ii) Infraorbital paraesthesia
    (iii) Cheek swelling

3. Oral cavity (10%)
    (i) Palatal swelling
    (ii) Palatal paraesthesia

4. Eye (5%)
    (i) Ocular paresis
    (ii) Proptosis
    (iii) Epiphora

5. Dental (4%)
    (i) Toothache
    (ii) Tooth loosening

PARANASAL SINUS TUMOURS PRESENT LATE. 20–50% ARE INCURABLE AT PRESENTATION

TUMOURS OF THE NASOPHARYNX

1. Benign — (rare) Juvenile angiofibroma

2. Malignant
    (i) Squamous cell carcinoma
    (ii) Lymphoma

Presentation of malignant nasopharyngeal tumours
    (i) Deafness due to secretory otitis media
    (ii) Cervical lymphadenopathy
    (iii) Diplopia due to sixth nerve palsy
    (iv) Nasal obstruction
    (v) Epistaxis
    (vi) Other cranial nerve involvement:
        a. II III IV (superior orbital fissure)
        b. V (foramen lacerum)
        c. IX X XI (jugular foramen)

Juvenile nasopharyngeal angiofibroma
Uncommon vascular benign tumour found in teenage boys.
- (i) Initial presentation
    - a. Nasal obstruction
    - b. Intermittent severe epistaxis
    - c. Deafness
- (ii) Late features
    - a. Nasal expansion, 'frog face'
    - b. Exophthalmos
- (iii) Treatment — Embolisation and excision

Rhinorrhoea

A DISCHARGE FROM THE NOSE WHICH MAY BE WATERY,
MUCOPURULENT OR BLOODSTAINED

CAUSES

1. Watery
   (i) Allergic rhinitis
   (ii) Vasomotor rhinitis
   (iii) Viral infection
   (iv) Cerebrospinal fluid

2. Mucopurulent
   (i) Bacterial rhinitis
   (ii) Sinusitis

3. Bloodstained
   (i) Severe rhinosinusitis
   (ii) Foreign body
   (iii) Malignant disease

CSF RHINORRHOEA

A watery discharge from the nose which contains glucose

1. Sites of CSF leaks into the nose
   (i) Cribriform plate
   (ii) Frontal sinus
   (iii) Ethmoid sinus
   (iv) Sphenoid sinus
   (v) Eustachian tube (CSF otorrhoea)

CSF rhinorrhoea is often dependent upon head position

2. Causes of CSF rhinorrhoea
    (i) Traumatic
        Anterior cranial fossa fractures
        Surgical
        a. Nasal — Polypectomy
                  Transeptal hypophysectomy
        b. Ethmoid sinus — Intranasal ethmoidectomy
                       Transethmoidal hypophysectomy
        c. Frontal sinus — Mucocoele
                     Osteoma
                     Osteoplastic flap
   (ii) Atraumatic
        a. Congenital anomalies
        b. Tumours eroding cribriform plate
        c. Spontaneous

PNEUMOCOCCAL MENINGITIS MAY BE THE PRESENTING
SYMPTOM OF CSF RHINORRHOEA. THE MORTALITY IS 20%

SINUSITIS

A. ACUTE SINUSITIS
Occurs in the paranasal sinuses in the following order of frequency:
    (i) Maxillary
   (ii) Ethmoids (children)
  (iii) Frontal
  (iv) Sphenoid (rare)
Can affect:
    (i) Single sinus
   (ii) Several sinuses (multisinusitis)
  (iii) All sinuses (pansinusitis)

1. Causes
    (i) Viral rhinitis with secondary bacterial
   (ii) infection
        a. *Haemophilus influenzae*
        b. *Staph. aureus*
        c. *Strep. pyogenes*
  (iii) Dental problems
        a. Apical abscess
        b. Extraction
        c. Oroantral fistula
   (iv) Swimming
        a. Ethmoiditis (children)
        b. Frontal sinusitis (adults)
    (v) Fractures involving sinuses

Table 13 Symptoms and signs of sinusitis

	Symptoms	Signs
Maxillary sinusitis	Persisting cold Cheek pain Purulent nasal discharge General malaise	Fever Cheek tenderness Pus in middle meatus and PNS Dental infection
Ethmoidal sinusitis	Pain behind eye Frontal headache Swelling of eyelids	Fever Periorbital cellulitis Pus in middle meatus
Frontal sinusitis	Periodic, severe frontal headache Swelling of upper eyelid	Fever Marked tenderness below supraorbital ridge

---

MAXILLARY SINUSITIS RARELY CAUSES CHEEK SWELLING UNLESS TOOTH ROOT INFECTION COEXISTS. IF ABSENT, A MAXILLARY CARCINOMA IS LIKELY

---

2. **Radiology**
   Sinus X-rays may show complete opacity or fluid levels

3. **Treatment**
   The aim of treatment is to encourage the re-opening of the obstructed sinus ostia

   Systemic antibiotics
   Nasal decongestants
   Analgesia

   | *Recovery delayed*
   ↓

   Antral washout/frontal sinus trephine and lavage

   | *Recovery delayed*
   ↓

   Intranasal antrostomy

B. CHRONIC SINUSITIS
Chronic inflammatory changes take place in the sinus mucosa as a result of the following cycle:

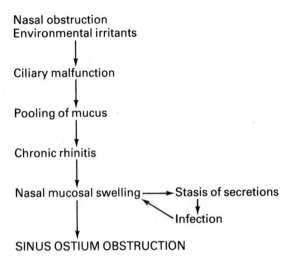

Nasal obstruction
Environmental irritants

↓

Ciliary malfunction

↓

Pooling of mucus

↓

Chronic rhinitis

↓

Nasal mucosal swelling ⟶ Stasis of secretions

↓

Infection

↓

SINUS OSTIUM OBSTRUCTION

1. Clinical picture
    (i) Severe pain is rare
   (ii) Dull facial ache
  (iii) Lethargy
  (iv) Symptoms of secondary infection
       a. Recurrent suppurative otitis media
       b. Serous otitis media
       c. Granular pharyngitis
       d. Chronic laryngitis
   (v) Acute exacerbations

2. Treatment
Local nasal or systemic decongestants may help in less severe cases but surgery is usually necessary

  (i) Maxillary   Repeated antral washouts

↓

Intranasal antrostomy

↓

Radical antrostomy and removal of antral mucosa (Caldwell-Luc operation)

(ii) Ethmoid   Eliminate maxillary sinus infection ± intranasal
                    polypectomy

                            ↓

                    External ethmoidectomy

(iii) Frontal   Eliminate maxillary sinus infection and causes
                    of fronto-nasal duct obstruction
                    (polyps, deviated septum)

                            ↓

                    Fronto-ethmoidectomy

                            ↓

                    Frontal sinus obliteration
                    (rarely performed)

C. COMPLICATIONS OF SINUS DISEASE

These are rare. They usually occur during acute exacerbations of
chronic fronto-ethmoidal sinusitis.

1. Orbital cellulitis
2. Mucocoele of frontal sinus
3. Osteomyelitis of frontal bone
4. Intracranial suppuration:
     (i) Extradural and subdural abscess
    (ii) Meningitis
   (iii) Cavernous sinus thrombosis
   (iv) Cerebral abscess

Rhinitis

INFLAMMATION OF THE MUCOSA OF THE NASAL FOSSAE

ACUTE

1. Viral
     (i) Common cold
    (ii) Influenza
   (iii) Exanthemata
2. Bacterial

CHRONIC

1. Infective
   (i) Non-specific
       Associated sinusitis,
       tonsillitis, adenoidal hypertrophy
  (ii) Specific
       a. TB
       b. Syphilis/yaws
       c. Fungal
       d. Diphtheria
       e. Leprosy

2. Non-infective
   (i) Allergic
       a. Seasonal — Pollens
       b. Perennial — Housedust
  (ii) Non-allergic
       a. Vasomotor
       b. Atrophic
       c. Hypertrophic — Rhinitis medicamentosa

RHINITIS: DEFINITIONS

1. Allergic rhinitis
A syndrome of watery rhinorrhoea, sneezing, nasal obstruction and watering, itchy eyes occurring in response to a specific allergen. The diagnosis is confirmed by positive skin testing

2. Vasomotor rhinitis
A syndrome of watery rhinorrhoea, intermittent nasal obstruction, a post nasal drip and paroxysmal sneezing. It results from a disturbance of the vasomotor control normally responsible for producing cyclical shrinkage and swelling of the nasal mucosa. It may be provoked by changes of humidity and temperature or non-specific atmospheric irritants. Endocrine and emotional factors may also play a part

3. Atrophic rhinitis (Ozaena)
A condition of unknown aetiology in which the nasal mucosa becomes sclerotic and the nasal fossae obstructed by crusts which produce an offensive smell. It may follow excessive surgery to the inferior turbinates

4. Rhinitis medicamentosa
Topical vasoconstrictors used for persisting nasal obstruction eventually produce rebound engorgement and permanent mucosal oedema which is unresponsive to further vasoconstrictors

Epistaxis

HAEMORRHAGE FROM THE NOSE

1. **Idiopathic**
   The commonest cause

2. **Local causes**
   (i) Traumatic
       a. Nose picking
       b. Foreign bodies
       c. Nasal surgery
       d. Fractures — Nasal bones
                       Sinuses
                       Base of skull
   (ii) Inflammatory
       a. Infective rhinitis
       b. Atrophic rhinitis
       c. Sinusitis
   (iii) Neoplastic
       a. Nose — Bleeding polypus of septum
                 Squamous carcinoma
       b. Sinuses — Squamous carcinoma
       c. Nasopharynx — Juvenile angiofibroma

3. **General causes**
   (i) Systemic hypertension
   (ii) Venous engorgement
       a. SVC obstruction
       b. Right heart failure
   (iii) Haematological and vascular
       a. Atherosclerosis
       b. Osler-Weber-Rendu
       c. Other vessel abnormalities
       d. Coagulation defects
       e. Thrombocytopenia
   (iv) Drugs
       a. Anticoagulants
       b. Salicylates

COMMONEST TYPES OF EPISTAXIS

1. Local

Spontaneous epistaxis from
Little's area in children
and adolescents

↓

Anterior nasal
haemorrhage

2. General

Hypertension in the
elderly

↓

Posterior nasal
haemorrhage

EPISTAXIS HAS AN ASSOCIATED MORTALITY. HYPOVOLAEMIC
SHOCK AND MYOCARDIAL INFARCTION MAY OCCUR,
ESPECIALLY IN THE ELDERLY

MANAGEMENT OF EPISTAXIS

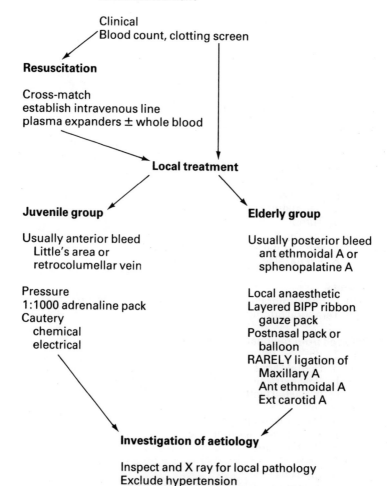

Initial assessment

Clinical
Blood count, clotting screen

Resuscitation

Cross-match
establish intravenous line
plasma expanders ± whole blood

Local treatment

Juvenile group

Usually anterior bleed
   Little's area or
   retrocolumellar vein

Pressure
1:1000 adrenaline pack
Cautery
   chemical
   electrical

Elderly group

Usually posterior bleed
   ant ethmoidal A or
   sphenopalatine A

Local anaesthetic
Layered BIPP ribbon
   gauze pack
Postnasal pack or
   balloon
RARELY ligation of
   Maxillary A
   Ant ethmoidal A
   Ext carotid A

Investigation of aetiology

Inspect and X ray for local pathology
Exclude hypertension
Exclude bleeding tendency
   and haematological abnormalities

Facial pain

CAUSES

1. Local
- (i) Facial lesions
  - a. Inflammation
  - b. Abscess
  - c. Haematoma
  - d. Tumour
- (ii) Nerve trauma
  - a. Infraorbital during Caldwell Luc
  - b. Ext nasal following nasal injury

2. Vascular
- (i) Periodic migrainous neuralgia, 'cluster headache'
- (ii) Temporal arteritis

3. Referred from regional structures
- (i) Teeth
  - a. Dental caries
  - b. Post extraction syndrome
  - c. Impacted teeth
- (ii) Nose
  - a. Mucosal congestion
  - b. Ant ethmoidal syndrome
  - c. Septal spurs
- (iii) Sinuses
  - a. Sinusitis
  - b. Tumours
- (iv) Eye
  - a. Iritis
  - b. Glaucoma
- (v) TM Joint
  - a. Dental malocclusion
  - b. Osteoarthritis
  - c. Bruxism
- (vi) Cerv Spine — Spondylosis

4. Specific neuralgias
- (i) Trigeminal
- (ii) Glossopharyngeal
- (iii) Post-herpetic

5. Muscle spasm – Secondary to — Malocclusion
Headache
6. Atypical facial neuralgia
- (i) Depression
- (ii) Conversion hysteria

DENTAL PROBLEMS ARE THE COMMONEST CAUSE OF FACIAL PAIN

TRIGEMINAL NEURALGIA

1. Primary — Tic douloureux
- (i) Features
  - a. Pain — Unilateral
    Severe
    Paroxysmal
    Trigeminal distribution
    Precipitated by sensory stimuli (Trigger zones)
  - b. No motor or sensory loss
  - c. Pain free between attacks
- (ii) Treatment
  - a. Medical — Carbamazepine
  - b. Surgical — Trigeminal ganglion injection
    Sensory root section in middle fossa

2. Secondary — Due to pressure from neighbouring pathology
- (i) Intracranial
  - a. Acoustic neuroma
  - b. Brain stem lesions — Multiple sclerosis
    Syringobulbia
    Arterial thrombosis
    Medullary tumours
- (ii) Extracranial
  - a. Nasopharyngeal carcinoma
  - b. Maxillary and mandibular tumours
  - c. Dental infection

PART THREE

The larynx, pharynx and neck

Anatomy

THE INVESTING FASCIAS OF THE NECK

1. Deep cervical fascia
This completely encircles the neck. It lies deep to the platysma muscle and splits to enclose the trapezius and sternomastoid muscles and the parotid and submandibular glands

2. Prevertebral fascia
This lies on the prevertebral musculature. The brachial plexus and subclavian artery lie deep to it and aquire a sheath from it which becomes the axillary sheath

3. Pretracheal fascia
This extends from the hyoid to the aortic arch and envelopes the thyroid gland. It fuses loosely laterally with the carotid sheath

4. Carotid sheath
This encloses the common carotid artery, the internal jugular vein and the vagus nerve

THE PHARYNX

The pharynx is a muscular tube, incomplete anteriorly, which conducts food and air to the stomach and lungs respectively. It extends from the skull base to the cricoid cartilage. It has openings anteriorly with the nose, the oral cavity and the larynx

The pharynx may be subdivided into
1. Nasopharynx above the soft palate
2. Oropharynx from the soft palate to the hyoid bone
3. Hypopharynx from the hyoid to the inferior border of the cricoid cartilage

The superior, middle and inferior constrictor muscles make up the main bulk of the pharyngeal musculature. These overlap each other from below upwards. The inferior constrictor comprises two distinct portions: the thyropharyngeus and cricopharyngeus

The glossopharyngeal and vagus nerves respectively provide the sensory and motor supply to the pharynx

THE LARYNX

The larynx is a cartilaginous framework completed by muscles, fibrous membranes and ligaments. The boundaries are:
1. Above — the laryngeal inlet made up of the free edge of the epiglottis, aryepiglottic folds, arytenoids and inter-arytenoid band
2. Below — the inferior border of the cricoid cartilage.
The free edge of the true vocal cord each side encloses an area called the glottis, with the supraglottis above and the subglottis below

1. **Cartilages**
    (i) Unpaired
        a. Thyroid
        b. Cricoid
        c. Epiglottis
    (ii) Paired
        a. Arytenoids
        b. Corniculates
        c. Cuneiforms

2. **Muscles**
    (i) Intrinsic
        a. Abductors — Posterior cricoarytenoids
        b. Adductors — Lateral cricoarytenoids
                        Interarytenoids
                        Thyroarytenoids
        c. Tensors — Cricothyroids
                      Vocalis
    (ii) Extrinsic
        a. Stylopharyngeus
        b. Palatopharyngeus
        c. Sternothyroid
        d. Thyrohyoid

Movement of the vocal cords results from rotation or sliding of the arytenoids on the cricoid cartilages brought about by the intrinsic muscles of the larynx

3. **Nerve supply**

   Motor: all the intrinsic muscles of the larynx are supplied by the recurrent laryngeal nerves EXCEPT the cricothyroids which are innervated by the external branches of the superior laryngeal nerves

   Sensory
   - (i) Supraglottis — Internal branches of superior laryngeal nerve
   - (ii) Glottis and subglottis — Recurrent laryngeal nerves

Physiology

SWALLOWING

Deglutition is a brainstem reflex controlled by a centre in the medulla. The reflex occurs in three stages, only the first of which is voluntary.

1. Oral stage
   The bolus is propelled back into the oropharynx by the contraction of mylohyoid which raises the floor of the mouth.

2. Pharyngeal stage
   On reaching the posterior pharyngeal wall, the bolus triggers off
   (i) Closure of the postnasal space by the soft palate
   (ii) Closure of the oral cavity by the faucial pillars and tongue
   (iii) Closure of the laryngeal inlet and cessation of respiration

3. Oesophageal stage
This consists of consecutive pressure changes in three zones
   (i) Relaxation of the pharyngo-oesophageal junction
   (ii) Generation of a peristaltic wave of contraction down the oesophagus
   (iii) Relaxation of the oesophago-gastric junction

FUNCTIONS OF THE LARYNX

1. Protection of the lower airway
2. Provision of a vibratory mechanism for phonation
3. Respiration

4. Voice production
This requires
   (i) Respiratory "bellows" to provide high subglottic pressure
   (ii) Vocal cords which provide a vibratory mechanism and a means of changing pitch
   (iii) Resonators
      a. Oral cavity
      b. Pharynx
      c. Nose
Theories of vocal cord vibration
   (i) Aerodynamic — Vocal cord vibration passive and depends on a high subglottic air pressure
   (ii) Neuromuscular — Cords vibrate as result of intrinsic muscle contraction (thought unlikely)

Sore throat

INFLAMMATORY

1. Infective
    (i) Tonsillitis
    (ii) Pharyngitis
    (iii) 2° to sinusitis
    (iv) Neck abscess
        a. Quinsy
        b. Parapharyngeal
        c. Retropharyngeal

2. Non-infective
    (i) Tobacco, alcohol
    (ii) Apthous ulcers
    (iii) Voice abuse
    (iv) Acid reflux
    (v) Foreign body abrasions
    (vi) Burns and corrosives

NON-INFLAMMATORY

1. Malignancy
    (i) Oropharynx
    (ii) Hypopharynx

2. Blood dyscrasias
    (i) Agranulocytosis
    (ii) Leukaemia

3. Neuralgia — Glossopharyngeal

ACUTE INFECTIVE PHARYNGITIS AND TONSILLITIS

1. Viral
- (i) Parainfluenza
- (ii) Adenovirus
- (iii) Rhinovirus
- (iv) Prodrome
    - a. Glandular fever
    - b. Measles
    - c. Typhoid

2. Bacterial
- (i) ß haemolytic *Streptococcus*
- (ii) *Strep. pneumoniae*
- (iii) *Haemophilus influenzae*
- (iv) *Gonococcus*
- (v) Secondary syphilis
- (vi) Diphtheria (rare)

3. Fungal
- (i) *Candida*
- (ii) *Actinomyces* (rare)

CHRONIC PHARYNGITIS AND TONSILLITIS

> THIS IS THE COMMONEST CAUSE OF CHRONIC SORE THROAT IN ADULTS

1. Predisposing factors
- (i) Chronic sinus infection with postnasal drip
- (ii) Nasal obstruction
- (iii) Voice overuse
- (iv) Smoking
- (v) Chronic cough and throat clearing
- (vi) Regular spirit drinking
- (vii) Infected teeth and gums
- (viii) Emotional and psychological problems

2. Symptoms
- (i) General discomfort in the throat
- (ii) Voice fatigue
- (iii) Repeated need to clear throat

3. Signs
- (i) Generalised erythema of oropharynx
- (ii) Lymphoid follicles on posterior pharyngeal wall
- (iii) Prominent lateral pharyngeal lymphoid bands
- (iv) Accompanying infection in tonsils

(v) Poor dentition
(vi) Rhinosinusitis

4. Treatment

AVOID INDISCRIMINATE USE OF ANTIBIOTICS
(i) Remove predisposing cause
(ii) Cautery/cryosurgery to lateral pharyngeal bands
(iii) Tonsillectomy may be indicated

CONSIDER THE POSSIBILITY OF SYPHILIS AND TB

SORE THROAT IN THE ADULT

1. History
(i) Acute or chronic
(ii) Fever
(iii) Dental caries
(iv) Spitting blood
(v) Smoking
(vi) Alcohol
(vii) Nasal obstruction
(viii) Nasal discharge
(ix) Earache
(x) Chronic cough
(xi) General health
(xii) Exposure to irritants

2. Examination
(i) Ears — Associated otitis media
(ii) Nose
   a. Deviated nasal septum
   b. Nasal polyps
   c. Rhinitis
(iii) PNS — Pus from infected sinus
(iv) Neck — Cervical nodes
   a. Tonsillitis
   b. Glandular fever
   c. Brucellosis
   d. Toxoplasmosis
   e. Metastatic
   f. Lymphoma
(v) Throat
   a. Oropharynx — Inflamed tonsils
                    Enlarged tonsils — Bilateral
                                       Unilateral
                    Prominent lateral bands
   b. Hypopharynx — Exclude malignancy

3. Investigations
- (i) Blood
    - a. Full blood count
    - b. Paul-Bunnell
    - c. Viral titres
    - d. Toxoplasma titres
    - e. *Brucella* titres
- (ii) X-Rays
    - a. Sinuses
    - b. Lateral neck
    - c. Chest
- (iii) Microbiology
    - a. Throat swab
    - b. Nasal swab
- (iv) Biopsy — ALL CASES OF UNILATERAL ENLARGED TONSILS

SORE THROAT IN THE CHILD

> THE COMMONEST CAUSES ARE VIRAL PHARYNGITIS AND ACUTE TONSILLITIS

ACUTE TONSILLITIS

1. Symptoms
- (i) Sore throat
- (ii) Dysphagia
- (iii) Fever
- (iv) Malaise
- (v) Abdominal pain
- (vi) Earache

2. Signs
- (i) Swollen exudative tonsils
- (ii) Pyrexia
- (iii) Furred tongue
- (iv) Foetor
- (v) Cervical lymphadenopathy

3. Additional clinical signs which may denote complications or another diagnosis
- (i) Rash — Exanthemata
- (ii) Bruising/Bleeding — Agranulocytosis/leukaemia
- (iii) Trismus — Peritonsillar abscess (quinsy)
- (iv) Stridor — Acute laryngeal oedema
- (v) Neck swelling — Parapharyngeal abscess
- (vi) Earache — Acute otitis media
- (vii) Arthropathy — Rheumatic fever
- (viii) Oedema — Glomerulonephritis

> THE ß HAEMOLYTIC STREPTOCOCCUS IS FREQUENTLY
> RESPONSIBLE BUT A VIRUS IS OFTEN THE PRIMARY CAUSE
>
> ACUTE TONSILLITIS IN CHILDREN IS FREQUENTLY RECURRENT

TONSILLECTOMY

1. Indications
- (i) Absolute
  - a. Sleep apnoea syndrome
  - b. Unilateral enlarged tonsil
- (ii) Relative
  - a. Recurrent acute bacterial tonsillitis
  - b. Chronic tonsillitis/pharyngitis
  - c. Quinsy
  - d. Recurrent otitis media
  - e. Recurrent chest infection associated with tonsillar infection
  - f. Recurrent systemic complications of ß haemolytic *Streptococcus* infection

> LARGE TONSILS ARE NOT IN THEMSELVES AN INDICATION FOR
> TONSILLECTOMY
>
> ALTHOUGH TONSILS AND ADENOIDS ARE OFTEN REMOVED
> SIMULTANEOUSLY, THE INDICATIONS FOR SURGERY IN EACH
> CASE SHOULD BE CONSIDERED SEPARATELY

2. Complications
- (i) Peroperative
  - a. Trauma to teeth, lips and tongue
  - b. Dislocation of TM joint
  - c. Cervical spine injury from hyperextension
- (ii) Immediate post-op
  - a. Reactionary haemorrhage — Slipped ligature
                                   Rise in BP
  - b. Airway obstruction
- (iii) Early
  - a. Secondary haemorrhage (classically Day 5–10) — infection and separation of slough
  - b. Referred otalgia (very common)
  - c. Otitis media
  - d. Oedema of soft palate and uvula
  - e. Local sepsis → cervical glands
  - f. Pneumonia from blood inhalation (rare)
- (iv) Late — Scarring and shortening of soft palate → rhinolalia operta

ADENOIDS

There is a physiological enlargement of the adenoid pad between 3 and 7 years of age

1. Symptoms and signs of the pathological adenoid
   (i) The hypertrophied adenoid
     a. Nasal obstruction and mouth breathing — Adenoid facies
                                         Snoring
                                         Sleep apnoea
     b. Eustachian tube obstruction — Secretory otitis media
                                        Deafness
  (ii) The inflamed adenoid
     a. Nasal discharge
     b. Post-nasal drip
     c. Cough
     d. Sinusitis
     e. Chronic suppurative and non-suppurative otitis media
     f. Cervical lymphadenopathy
     g. Retropharyngeal abscess

2. Indications for adenoidectomy
   (i) Sleep apnoea syndrome
     a. Night apnoeic episodes
     b. Poor feeding/failure to thrive
     c. Pulmonary hypertension/right heart failure
  (ii) Nasal obstruction
 (iii) Persisting deafness due to glue ear
 (iv) Recurrent sinusitis
  (v) Recurrent chest infection
 (vi) Recurrent acute otitis media

ADENOIDECTOMY SHOULD NOT BE PERFORMED IF A
SUBMUCOUS CLEFT PALATE OR BIFID UVULA IS PRESENT

Dysphagia

DIFFICULTY IN SWALLOWING

CAUSES

1. Congenital
- (i) Tracheo-oesophageal fistula
- (ii) Dysphagia lusoria (aberrant subclavian A)
- (iii) Congenital hiatus hernia
- (iv) Congenital oesophageal stricture

2. Acquired
- (i) Central
  - a. Neurological — Motor neurone disease
      Multiple sclerosis
      Myaesthenia gravis
      Bilateral vagal palsy
  - b. Psychological — Globus hystericus
- (ii) Pre-oesophageal
  - a. Infective — Acute tonsillitis
      Chronic pharyngitis
      Quinsy
      Parapharyngeal abscess
      Ludwig's angina
  - b. Neoplastic — Oral cavity, oro-hypopharynx, larynx,
      parapharyngeal space
- (iii) Oesophageal
  - a. Infective — Monilial oesophagitis
  - b. Neoplastic — Benign leiomyoma
      Malignant carcinoma
  - c. Inflammatory — Oesophagitis, stricture, radiotherapy
  - d. Neurological — Achalasia, diffuse spasm
  - e. Extrinsic — Mediastinal glands, neoplasms (bronchus,
      thyroid, stomach) osteophytes, aortic
      aneurysm,
  - f. Miscellaneous — Pharyngeal pouch, scleroderma,
      foreign body, Plummer-Vinson

INVESTIGATION OF DYSPHAGIA

> **EXCLUDE MALIGNANCY IF DYSPHAGIA REMAINS UNDIAGNOSED FOR MORE THAN ONE MONTH**

1. **History**
   - (i) Duration
   - (ii) Site
   - (iii) Intermittent or constant
   - (iv) Progressive
   - (v) Fluids or solids
   - (vi) Regurgitation or aspiration
   - (vii) Dyspepsia
   - (viii) Smoking and alcohol

2. **Examination**
   - (i) General — Weight loss, anaemia, hydration
   - (ii) Oral cavity
   - (iii) Indirect laryngoscopy
   - (iv) Nose and post-nasal space
   - (v) Neck
   - (vi) Chest
   - (vii) Abdomen
   - (viii) Neurological

3. **Investigation**
   - (i) Blood
     - a. Full blood count
     - b. Serum iron and TIBC
     - c. B_{12} and folate
     - d. Urea and electrolytes, liver function
   - (ii) Radiology
     - a. Soft tissue lateral neck
     - b. Chest
     - c. Barium swallow + cineradiography
     - d. Barium meal
   - (iii) Surgical
     - a. Panendoscopy
     - b. Oesophago-gastroscopy
     - c. Oesophageal pressure studies

The choice of investigation is determined by the clinical findings. A diagnosis of globus hystericus or psychogenic dysphagia should only be made after the patient has been fully investigated and organic pathology excluded

> **ENDOSCOPY IS MANDATORY IN EVERY CASE WHERE THE DIAGNOSIS IS IN DOUBT**

CARCINOMA OF THE OESOPHAGUS

1. Predisposing factors
  (i) Males > females
  (ii) Alcohol and tobacco
  (iii) Achalasia
  (iv) Plummer-Vinson syndrome
  (v) Reflux oesophagitis
  (vi) Geographical (Far East)

Table 14

Site	Incidence	Histology
Upper 1/3	25%	Squamous carcinoma
Middle 1/3	50%	Squamous carcinoma
Lower 1/3	25%	Adenocarcinoma

2. Treatment
  (i) Upper 1/3 — Radiotherapy or 3-stage total oesophagectomy
  (ii) Middle 1/3 — Radiotherapy or 2 or 3-stage total oesophagectomy
  (iii) Lower 1/3 — Surgery
      a. Below diaphragm — 1-stage oesophago-gastrectomy
      b. Above diaphragm — 2-stage oesophagectomy

ADENOCARCINOMA OF THE OESOPHAGUS IS RADIORESISTANT

At presentation most tumours are advanced and only suitable for palliative treatment. Swallowing may be temporarily maintained by intubation of the tumour. The most commonly used tubes are: Mousseau-Barbin, Celestin, Souttar, Nottingham

THE FIVE-YEAR SURVIVAL RATE IS 2%

ACHALASIA

A neuromuscular disorder of the lower end of the oesophagus which fails to relax normally on swallowing

1. Clinical features
  (i) Dysphagia — Initially intermittent, later constant
  (ii) Retrosternal discomfort
  (iii) Regurgitation and aspiration pneumonia
  (iv) Weight loss

2. **Radiological features**
   Gross dilatation of the proximal oesophagus gives a
   characteristic appearance on barium swallow

3. **Treatment**
   Heller's cardiomyotomy
   Dilatation of narrowed segment with bougies or a hydrostatic bag

RUPTURE OF THE OESOPHAGUS

1. **Causes**
     (i) Severe vomiting
    (ii) Traumatic
         a. Foreign body
         b. Surgical instrumentation
         c. Open neck trauma
   (iii) Caustic ingestion
    (iv) Radiotherapy
     (v) Peptic ulceration
    (vi) Neoplasm

2. **Clinical presentation**
     (i) Pain
    (ii) Dyspnoea
   (iii) Surgical emphysema in the neck
    (iv) Shock

3. **Radiology**
     (i) Barium swallow
    (ii) May be hydropneumothorax on chest X-ray

PLUMMER VINSON SYNDROME

1. **Clinical features**
     (i) Almost exclusively middle aged women
    (ii) Progressive dysphagia
   (iii) Features of iron deficiency
         a. Microcytic anaemia
         b. Glossitis and angular stomatitis
         c. Koilonychia
    (iv) Post-cricoid web (70%)
     (v) Achlorhydria (70%)
    (vi) Pre-malignant (Post-cricoid carcinoma in 10%)

2. **Management**
     (i) Correction of iron deficiency anaemia
    (ii) Oesophagoscopy and dilatation of any stricture
   (iii) Long-term follow up

CARCINOMA OF THE HYPOPHARYNX

Almost all are squamous cell carcinomas

1. Site
    (i) Piriform fossa (55%)
    (ii) Post-cricoid (40%)
    (iii) Posterior pharyngeal wall (5%)

2. Presentation
    (i) Dysphagia
    (ii) Hoarseness
    (iii) Pain (local or referred to ear)
    (iv) Cervical lymphadenopathy
    (v) Weight loss and cachexia

PRESENTATION IS LATE, PROGNOSIS IS POOR

3. Treatment
    (i) Radiotherapy — Tumours confined to the hypopharynx
                           without palpable nodes
    (ii) Surgery
        a. Advanced tumours with spread outside hypopharynx OR
          recurrence after radiotherapy
        b. Partial or total pharyngolaryngectomy with
          reconstruction of the pharynx. Radical neck dissection is
          performed for involved lymph nodes

LESIONS OF THE ORAL CAVITY

1. Swellings of the floor of the mouth
    (i) Congenital
        a. Dermoid
        b. Lymphangioma
        c. Haemangioma
    (ii) Acquired
        a. Inflammatory — Ludwig's angina, dental abscess
        b. Cysts — Ranula, mucous retention cyst
        c. Calculi — Submandibular duct
        d. Neoplastic — Benign — Fibroma,
                              Lymphangioma
                              Haemangioma
                    Malignant — Squamous carcinoma
                                Minor salivary gland tumour

2. Swellings of the tongue
  (i) Congenital
   a. Lingual thyroid, lymphangioma
   b. Haemangioma, cretinism
   c. Down's syndrome
  (ii) Acquired
   a. Allergic — Angioneurotic oedema
   b. Iatrogenic — Surgery
   c. Neoplastic — Benign — Fibroma
                                    Granular cell myoblastoma
                      Malignant — Squamous cell carcinoma
   d. Endocrine — Acromegaly

3. Oral ulceration

> MUCH THE COMMONEST CAUSE IS APHTHOUS ULCERATION

  (i) Inflammatory
   a. Infective — Bacterial — Vincent's angina
                               Tuberculosis
                               Syphilis
                               Cancrum oris
                    Viral — *Herpes*
                            Exanthemata
                    Fungal — *Candida*
   b. Non-infective — Traumatic — Ill fitting dentures
                                          Cheek biting
                                          Burns
                          Radiotherapy

  (ii) Haematological
   a. Leukaemia
   b. Agranulocytosis
  (iii) Neoplastic — Malignant ulcer
  (iv) Autoimmune
   a. Aphthous
   b. Behçet's
   c. Reiter's
   d. Stevens-Johnson
  (v) Skin conditions
   a. Pemphigoid
   b. Pemphigus vulgaris
   c. Lichen planus
  (vi) Vitamin deficiency
   a. C (Scurvy)
   b. Riboflavin
   c. Nicotinic acid

Stridor

NOISY BREATHING DUE TO NARROWING OF THE LUMEN OF
LARYNX OR TRACHEA

CAUSES OF STRIDOR IN ADULTS

1. Infective
   (i) Laryngotracheitis
   (ii) Neck space abscess
      a. Parapharyngeal
      b. Retropharyngeal

2. Neoplastic
   (i) Larynx — Squamous carcinoma
   (ii) Trachea
      a. Intrinsic — 1° tumour (rare)
      b. Extrinsic — Carcinoma bronchus, oesophagus
                      Thyroid lesions
                      2° mediastinal nodes

3. Traumatic
   (i) Foreign bodies
   (ii) Complications of surgery and intubation
      a. Oedema
      b. Glottic webs
      c. Intubation granuloma
      d. Subglottic stenosis
      e. Bilateral recurrent laryngeal nerve palsy

4. Allergic — Angioneurotic oedema

```
WHEN STRIDOR IS PRESENT, COMPLETE RESPIRATORY
OBSTRUCTION MAY RAPIDLY SUPERVENE AND REQUIRE
EMERGENCY TRACHEOSTOMY
```

CAUSES OF STRIDOR IN CHILDREN

1. Congenital
(i) Laryngomalacia
(ii) Cysts
(iii) Webs
(iv) Tumours
(v) Subglottic stenosis
(vi) Vocal cord paralysis

2. Acquired
(i) Infective
    a. Acute epiglottitis
    b. Acute laryngotracheo-bronchitis ("croup")
    c. Acute laryngitis
(ii) Neoplastic — Multiple papillomatosis
(iii) Foreign body

STRIDOR IN CHILDREN SHOULD NOT BE ATTRIBUTED TO LARYNGOMALACIA WITHOUT THOROUGH INVESTIGATION

ACUTE EPIGLOTTITIS AND ACUTE LARYNGO-TRACHEO-BRONCHITIS (LTB; CROUP)

Acute epiglottitis is usually caused by *Haemophilus influenzae* type B. Laryngo-tracheo-bronchitis is usually viral, caused by the parainfluenza, respiratory syncitial or measles viruses. Clinical differentiation between the two groups often proves difficult. The following are GENERALISATIONS but may be helpful

1. Epiglottitis
(i) Age 3–6 years
(ii) Localised supraglottic infection
(iii) Rapid course
(iv) Croupy cough less common
(v) Child sits up with mouth open and chin forward

2. LTB ("Croup")
(i) Age 6/12 to 3 years
(ii) Laryngeal, tracheal and bronchial exudates and crusts
(iii) More protracted course
(iv) Croupy cough usual
(v) Child tends to lie down

EXAMINATION OF THE THROAT IN CASES OF EPIGLOTTITIS MAY PRECIPITATE LARYNGEAL OBSTRUCTION AND SUDDEN RESPIRATORY ARREST

TRACHEOSTOMY

AN OPENING CREATED IN THE ANTERIOR WALL OF THE TRACHEA
TO ESTABLISH AN AIRWAY

Whenever possible, an endotracheal tube should be passed by an
experienced anaesthetist. Emergency tracheostomy is performed
only if intubation proves impossible. Elective tracheostomy is
performed if endotracheal intubation is necessary for more than 5–7
days, since prolonged intubation carries its own morbidity (*qv*)

INDICATIONS

1. **Relief of acute airway obstruction**
   (i) Above the larynx
      a. Trauma — Facial fractures
                        Soft tissue swelling
      b. Infection — Ludwigs angina
      c. Foreign body
      d. Tumours
   (ii) In the larynx ⎫ CAUSES AS FOR STRIDOR
   (iii) Below the larynx ⎭

2. **Protection of the tracheobronchial tree**
   Against — Inhalation of saliva, food, gastric contents or
                  blood

   Causes

   a. Coma
   b. Polyneuritis
   c. Myaesthenia gravis
   d. Tetanus
   e. Bulbar and pseudobulbar palsies

3. **Respiratory insufficiency**
   (i) Acute
      a. Flail chest
      b. Overwhelming infection
   (ii) Chronic
      a. Neuromuscular weakness
      b. Musculoskeletal deformity

In respiratory insufficiency, tracheostomy is required:
   to permit intermittent positive pressure ventilation or
   to allow suction of stagnant bronchial secretions

SUMMARY OF THE FUNCTIONS OF A TRACHEOSTOMY

1. Bypasses obstruction
2. Permits intermittent positive pressure ventilation
3. Decreases anatomical dead space by 10–50%
4. Decreases airways resistance
5. Protects against aspiration
6. Allows frequent suction
7. Allows speech and swallowing in the conscious patient

COMMON TYPES OF TRACHEOSTOMY TUBE

1. Portex/silicone
      (i) Cuffed (low pressure, high volume)
      (ii) Uncuffed

2. Silver
    Negus/Chevalier Jackson
    a. Introducer
    b. Inner tube ± speaking valve
    c. Outer tube

Sizes
a. Women 30 or 33 FG
b. Men 33 or 35 FG

The largest tube which comfortably fits the tracheostomy should be used. This is usually ¾ diameter of the trachea

COMPLICATIONS OF TRACHEOSTOMY

1. Immediate
      (i) Haemorrhage
      (ii) Surgical trauma
          a. Oesophagus
          b. Recurrent laryngeal nerve
          c. Apex of lung
      (iii) Pneumothorax

2. Intermediate
      (i) Tracheobronchitis
      (ii) Tracheal erosion and haemorrhage
      (iii) Tube displacement
      (iv) Tube obstruction
      (v) Subcutaneous emphysema
      (vi) Aspiration and lung abscess

3. Late
   (i) Persistent tracheocutaneous fistula
   (ii) Laryngeal and tracheal stenosis
   (iii) Tracheomalacia
   (iv) Difficult decannulation
   (v) Tracheo — oesophageal fistula
   (vi) Tracheostomy scar

THE MORTALITY ASSOCIATED WITH TRACHEOSTOMY IS 1.6% IN ADULTS AND 5% IN CHILDREN

CRICOTHYROTOMY

An opening in the cricothyroid membrane

This may be performed in an emergency to establish an airway rapidly if the equipment and/or expertise necessary for tracheostomy are not immediately available

1. Advantage
   Minimum of equipment and surgical dissection necessary

2. Disadvantages
   (i) Narrow space; difficult to place tracheostomy tube without damage to cricoid, leading to perichondritis and stenosis
   (ii) Damage to vocal cords leading to voice change
   (iii) Perforation of cricothyroid artery leading to severe bleeding

Hoarseness

A ROUGHNESS OF THE VOICE RESULTING FROM AN
ABNORMALITY WITHIN THE LARYNX

CAUSES

1. **Congenital**
   - (i) Glottic web
   - (ii) Subglottic stenosis
   - (iii) Haemangioma
   - (iv) Cysts

2. **Acquired**
   - (i) Inflammatory
     - a. Infective laryngitis
     - b. Non-infective laryngitis
   - (ii) Neoplastic
     - a. Benign — Papillomas
     - b. Malignant — Squamous cell carcinoma
   - (iii) Traumatic
     - a. Intubation
     - b. External injury
   - (iv) Neurological — Vocal cord palsy
   - (v) Miscellaneous
     - a. Functional dysphonia
     - b. Myxoedema
     - c. Radiotherapy

INVESTIGATIONS

> EXCLUDE MALIGNANCY IF HOARSENESS PERSISTS FOR MORE
> THAN ONE MONTH

1. History
- (i) Recent respiratory tract infection
- (ii) Duration
- (iii) Intermittent or constant
- (iv) Smoking and alcohol
- (v) Dysphagia
- (vi) Associated nasal symptoms
- (vii) Associated pulmonary symptoms

2. Examination
- (i) Oral cavity
- (ii) Indirect laryngoscopy
- (iii) Nose and postnasal space
- (iv) Neck
- (v) Chest

3. Investigation
- (i) Blood
  - a. Full blood count
  - b. Thyroid function
  - c. VDRL/TPHA
- (ii) Radiology
  - a. Soft tissue lateral neck
  - b. Chest
  - c. Sinuses
  - d. Barium swallow
  - e. Laryngeal tomography
  - f. Base of skull tomography
- (iii) Surgical
  - a. Direct laryngoscopy and biopsy
  - b. Oesophagoscopy

The choice of investigation is determined by the clinical findings

> ENDOSCOPY IS MANDATORY IN EVERY CASE WHERE THE
> DIAGNOSIS IS IN DOUBT

LARYNGITIS

1. Causes
    (i) Acute
        a. Non-specific — Infective: viral, bacterial
                                   Traumatic: voice abuse
                                   Toxins: fumes, corrosives
        b. Specific — Diphtheria
    (ii) Chronic
        a. Non-specific — Infective: Secondary to chronic sinusitis
                                   or dental caries
                                   Traumatic — Voice abuse
                                   Toxins — Alcohol, tobacco, dusts,
                                   steroid inhalers
        b. Specific — Tuberculosis
                        Syphilis

Recurrent acute laryngitis may predispose to chronic laryngitis. There is often more than one predisposing factor involved in the aetiology of chronic non-specific laryngitis

2. Laryngeal appearances
    (i) Localised
        a. Vocal cord polyps
        b. Vocal cord nodules
    (ii) Generalised
        a. Hyperaemia
        b. Hypertrophy
        c. Oedema (Reinke's)

VOCAL CORD PALSY

THE COMMONEST CAUSES OF A VOCAL CORD PALSY

1. Malignant disease
2. Idiopathic
3. Surgical trauma

Vocal cord palsy is more common on the left due to the long intrathoracic course of the left recurrent laryngeal nerve

---

A VOCAL CORD PALSY MAY RESULT FROM LESIONS INVOLVING EITHER THE TRUNK OF THE VAGUS NERVE OR THE RECURRENT LARYNGEAL NERVE

---

1. Vagal palsies

THE VOCAL CORD IS HELD IN THE CADAVERIC POSITION MIDWAY
BETWEEN THE MIDLINE AND MODERATE ABDUCTION

(i) Causes
a. Bulbar palsies — Motor neurone disease
   Medullary tumours
   Posterior inferior cerebellar artery
   thrombosis
   Bulbar polio
b. Skull base lesions — Fractures
   Nasopharyngeal carcinoma
c. High neck lesions — Penetrating injury
   Tumours

(ii) Presentation
a. Unilateral palsy — Aspiration
   Hoarseness
b. Bilateral palsy — Severe aspiration
   Very weak voice

RECURRENT LARYNGEAL NERVE PALSY

THE VOCAL CORD IS HELD IN THE PARAMEDIAN POSITION

Causes

1. Neck
(i) Penetrating injury
(ii) Thyroid
  a. Multinodular goitre
  b. Carcinoma
  c. Thyroidectomy
(iii) Oesophagus — carcinoma
(iv) Glands
  a. 1° tumours
  b. 2° tumours
  c. Tuberculosis (rare)

2. Chest — (Left only)
(i) Mediastinal glands
(ii) Bronchial carcinoma
(iii) Oesophageal carcinoma
(iv) Tuberculosis
(v) Aortic aneurysm
(vi) Large left atrium

If all the investigations are negative, a provisional diagnosis of idiopathic vocal cord palsy is made. Regular follow up is imperative because a bronchial carcinoma may subsequently become apparent

LARYNGEAL TUMOURS

1. **Classification**
    - (i) Benign
        - a. Papilloma
        - b. Haemangioma
        - c. Chondroma
    - (ii) Malignant
        - a. Squamous cell carcinoma
        - b. Undifferentiated carcinoma

Primary malignant tumours of the larynx may arise in the supraglottis, glottis or subglottis. Advanced lesions may involve more than one of these regions

The most common extrinsic tumours to involve the larynx are carcinomas of the thyroid, hypopharynx and oesophagus

Virtually all cases of squamous cell carcinoma of the larynx occur in smokers

2. **Presentation**
    - (i) Hoarseness
    - (ii) Dry cough
    - (iii) Otalgia
    - (iv) Dysphagia
    - (v) Stridor
    - (vi) Lump in the neck

3. **Treatment**
    - (i) Radiotherapy — If tumour is
        - a. Confined to larynx
        - b. Cord is mobile
        - c. No palpable nodes
    - (ii) Surgery — Laryngectomy if
        - a. Spread outside larynx
        - b. Fixed cord
        - c. Recurrences after radiotherapy
        - d. + radical neck dissection if palpable nodes

Speech disorders

DYSPHASIA

Difficulty in the understanding or production of language. Results from damage to the dominant cerebral hemisphere, usually by cerebrovascular disease or tumour

1. Receptive (sensory) dysphasia
    Difficulty in comprehension of language
2. Expressive (motor) dysphasia
    Comprehension normal, but central production of language impaired
    Receptive and expressive dysphasia frequently occur together; in such cases, one type usually predominates

DYSARTHRIA

Difficulty in articulating and enunciating words correctly, due to disorders of the neuromuscular control of the muscles of articulation. Dysarthria may be classified in several ways; characteristics of the different forms are better learnt from clinical observation than from their description

1. **Spastic dysarthria**
    Upper motor neurone damage (pseudobulbar palsy). Lesions must be bilateral before there is significant dysarthria. Multiple sclerosis, motor neurone disease, upper brainstem tumours.
    Speech slurred and indistinct

2. **Rigid dysarthria**
    Extrapyramidal disease (usually Parkinsonism). Speech monotonous, words merge, inflection and accent absent

3. **Ataxic dysarthria**
    Cerebellar lesions. Speech irregular and slurred. Jerky variation of timing and volume

4. Bulbar dysarthria

Lower motor neurone damage. Often causes problems with individual words and sounds, others well preserved.

Tongue paralysis affects a large number of sounds and causes the most profound speech disturbance.

Palatal paralysis produces nasal speech. Consonants b, d, n, g, k cause difficulties.

Facial paralysis causes difficulty with labial consonants b, p, m, w

DYSLALIA

Abnormal articulation due to abnormalities of the tongue, lips, teeth or palate ("the peripheral speech apparatus")

DYSRHYTHMIA

Stammering. Disturbance of the normal rhythm of speech with sudden interruptions of flow and repetition of sounds. Rarely any other neurological abnormality detectable, but occasionally it is a manifestation of a mild dysphasia

Note also that cerebellar lesions affect respiratory muscles as well as articulatory musculature and disrupt rhythm

DYSPHONIA

Impairment of pitch, quality or loudness of voice due to abnormality within the larynx, its innervation or to psychogenic disorder. The term includes hoarseness (qv). Complete absence of phonation is termed aphonia. If the aphonic patient can cough normally a psychogenic origin should be suspected

---

A SPEECH PROBLEM MAY COMBINE TWO OR MORE OF THE ABOVE TYPES OF SPEECH DISORDER

MILESTONES IN SPEECH DEVELOPMENT

1. 9–15 months — First words spoken
2. 18 months — 20 word vocabulary
3. 24 months — Word combinations
4. 36 months — Sentences used

It is imperative to remember that deafness is a common cause of slow or faulty speech development in the child

> ALL CHILDREN WITH A SPEECH DISORDER SHOULD BE FULLY INVESTIGATED FOR HEARING LOSS

Mental retardation or social deprivation may present as a speech disorder

INVESTIGATIONS

1. History
  (i) Duration
  (ii) Developmental and speech milestones (children)
  (iii) Associated neurological symptoms
  (iv) Associated otological symptoms
  (v) Social and psychiatric history

2. Initial examination
  (i) Ears
  (ii) Oral cavity and pharynx
  (iii) Neurological system
  (iv) Clinical assessment of intelligence
  (v) Indirect laryngoscopy

3. Investigations and further examination
  (i) Blood
    a. Full blood count
    b. Thyroid function
  (ii) Radiological
    a. Soft tissue lateral neck
    b. Chest
    c. Skull
    d. Head CT scan
  (iii) Audiological — Investigations for deafness (*qv*)
  (iv) Surgical
    a. Direct laryngoscopy
    b. Nasendoscopy for palatal function
  (v) Behavioural & IQ testing

INVESTIGATIONS ARE DETERMINED BY THE CLINICAL FINDINGS

Lump in the neck

SUBMANDIBULAR TRIANGLE

1. Submandibular calculus
2. Submandibular sialectasis
3. Submandibular tumour
4. Metastatic node

MIDLINE SWELLINGS

1. Thyroid swelling
2. Thyroglossal cyst
3. Dermoid cyst
4. Laryngeal chondroma

POSTERIOR TRIANGLE

1. Lymphadenopathy
   - (i) Glandular fever
   - (ii) Rubella
   - (iii) Scalp infestation
   - (iv) Tuberculosis
   - (v) Toxoplasma/CMV
   - (vi) Lymphoma
2. Cervical rib

ANTERIOR TRIANGLE

1. Lymphadenopathy
   - (i) Non-specific infections, e.g.
     - a. Tonsillitis
     - b. Pharyngitis
     - c. Rhinosinusitis
     - d. Dental caries
     - e. Skin infections
     - f. Mouth ulcer
   - (ii) Tuberculosis

(iii) Metastatic nodes from head and neck
(iv) lymphoma
2. Branchial cyst
3. Carotid body tumour
4. Carotid aneurysm
5. Laryngocele
6. Pharyngeal pouch

SUPRACLAVICULAR FOSSA

1. Metastatic nodes — (bronchus & stomach commonest)
2. Pancoast tumours
3. Subclavian aneurysm

CONGENITAL CYSTS

	Thyroglossal cyst	Branchial cyst
Site	90% midline	66% on left (anterior triangle)
Moves on swallowing	Yes	No
External sinus	Only after previous surgery	Occasionally
Internal sinus	Invariably a track up into foramen caecum	Occasionally
Function	May be the only functioning thyroid Scan mandatory pre-op	None
Treatment	Sistrunk's operation, with removal of body of hyoid	Excise, with any sinus present

PHARYNGEAL POUCH

1. Clinical features
    (i) Usually elderly patients
    (ii) Dysphagia
    (iii) Choking ± regurgitation of food
    (iv) Recurrent chest infections
    (v) Typical appearance on barium swallow
    (vi) 90% occur on left (on right in left-handers)
2. Treatment
    (i) Oesophagoscopy to exclude malignancy in all cases
    (ii) Excision ± cricopharyngeal myotomy
    (iii) Dohlman's procedure: endoscopic diathermy division of party wall between pouch and oesophagus

NEOPLASTIC SALIVARY GLAND SWELLINGS

Salivary gland tumours may involve the parotid, submandibular, sublingual or minor salivary glands, the parotid being the most commonly affected. The smaller the gland the lower the overall incidence of tumour, but the higher the likelihood of any one tumour being malignant

1. Benign
   (i) Mixed parotid tumour (pleomorphic adenoma). 60% of parotid tumours. Notorious for tendency to recur, needs good margins of excision (superficial parotidectomy)
  (ii) Adenolymphoma (Warthin's tumour). Parotid only, 10% bilateral. Occurs in elderly men
 (iii) Haemangioma in children
 (iv) Lymphangioma in children

2. Malignant
   (i) Adenoid cystic carcinoma (cylindroma). Spreads perineurally. Late recurrence
  (ii) Adenocarcinoma. Occasionally may be a 2° from elsewhere
 (iii) Squamous cell carcinoma. Elderly. Aggressive. May be a 2°
 (iv) Arising in pleomorphic adenoma. Probably true malignant change in previously benign tumour

3. Intermediate
   (i) Mucoepidermoid tumour. High-grade type behaves like a squamous cell carcinoma
  (ii) Acinic cell carcinoma (rare). Virtually confined to parotid
 (iii) Oncocytoma (rare)

These tumours should be regarded with suspicion. It is often impossible to make histological distinction between benign and malignant tumours. They comprise 10% of submandibular and minor salivary gland tumours

NON-NEOPLASTIC SALIVARY GLAND ENLARGEMENT

1. Sialadenitis
    (i) Acute
        a. Viral — Mumps
                 CMV
        b. Bacterial — Poor oral hygiene
                     Dehydration
                     During DXT
    (ii) Recurrent acute
        a. Obstructive — Calculus
                     Stricture
        b. Non-obstructive — Cause unknown — Children 5–10
                                       Women menopause
    (iii) Chronic
        a. Tuberculosis
        b. Actinomycosis

2. Calculi — 80% submandibular

3. Cysts
    (i) Simple cysts (parotid)
    (ii) Mucous retention
    (iii) Ranula (sublingual)

4. Systemic disease
    (i) Alcoholism
    (ii) Pancreatitis
    (iii) Diabetes mellitus
    (iv) Acromegaly
    (v) Malnutrition

5. Sjogren's

6. Sarcoidosis — Heerfordt's syndrome

7. Mikulicz's syndrome
    (i) Leukaemia
    (ii) Lymphoma
    (iii) Tuberculosis
    (iv) Sarcoidosis

8. Drug induced
    (i) Phenothiazines
    (ii) Phenylbutazone

9. Allergic — Iodine

MANAGEMENT OF THE LUMP IN THE PAROTID

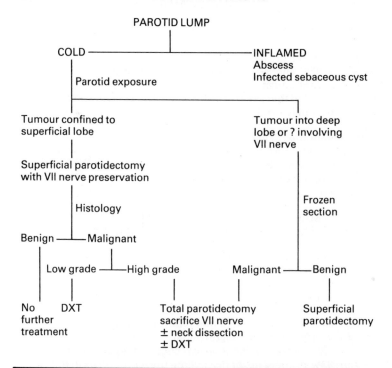

FACIAL NERVE PARALYSIS CARRIES AN ADVERSE PROGNOSIS.
THE INCIDENCE OF METASTASES IN SUCH CASES IS HIGH

A disparity of opinion exists in the management of malignant
tumours of the parotid, especially with regard to:
1. Sacrifice of the facial nerve if not clinically involved
2. Elective neck dissection
3. Post-operative radiotherapy
4. Use of aspiration cytology in diagnosis — Used in some centres
but can be misleading

MANAGEMENT OF THE SUSPECTED METASTATIC CERVICAL NODE WITH OCCULT PRIMARY

BIOPSY AT AN EARLY STAGE IS NOT RECOMMENDED

When metastatic disease is present in a node in the cervical chain, there is an 85% chance of the primary being found in the head and neck. The commonest sites are the nasopharynx (55%), tonsil, tongue base and thyroid. By contrast, metastatic supraclavicular nodes are usually from primaries below the clavicles

1. **Disadvantages of cervical node biopsy**
   May lead to tumour implantation in the skin. The 5-year survival is then considerably reduced. If the primary is not found as a consequence of an inadequate search, the potential survival is reduced

   THE PRIMARY SHOULD BE FOUND AND THE WHOLE AREA TREATED AS ONE WITHOUT PRIOR NODE BIOPSY

2. **Early biopsy is only recommended**
   (i) For children in whom neck masses are usually inflammatory or congenital
   (ii) For supraclavicular, rather than cervical, neck masses

3. **Success of investigation of metastatic cervical node**
   (i) 33% primary evident on initial investigation (see plan)
   (ii) 33% primary evident on investigation repeated later
   (iii) 33% primary never discovered (best prognosis in this group)

4. **Survival rates**
   (i) 60% alive and disease free at 1 year
   (ii) 15% alive and disease free at 5 years

THE SEARCH FOR THE OCCULT PRIMARY

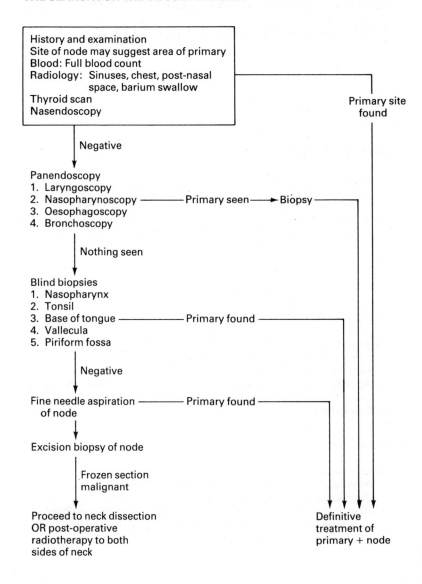

History and examination
Site of node may suggest area of primary
Blood: Full blood count
Radiology: Sinuses, chest, post-nasal
              space, barium swallow
Thyroid scan
Nasendoscopy

Primary site
found

Negative

Panendoscopy
1. Laryngoscopy
2. Nasopharynoscopy ————— Primary seen ——→ Biopsy ———
3. Oesophagoscopy
4. Bronchoscopy

Nothing seen

Blind biopsies
1. Nasopharynx
2. Tonsil
3. Base of tongue ————————— Primary found ———
4. Vallecula
5. Piriform fossa

Negative

Fine needle aspiration ————— Primary found ———
   of node

Excision biopsy of node

Frozen section
malignant

Proceed to neck dissection
OR post-operative
radiotherapy to both
sides of neck

Definitive
treatment of
primary + node

ENT manifestations of HIV infection and AIDS

CERVICAL LYMPHADENOPATHY

Causes
   (i) Uncomplicated lymphadenopathy, occuring with or without an infective focus in the upper aerodigestive tract
   (ii) Persistant generalised lymphadenopathy (PGL)
       This is enlargement of lymph nodes in two or more extra-inguinal sites lasting for more than 3 months
   (iii) B cell lymphoma
   (iv) Malignant involvement from a Kaposi's sarcoma or oral cavity carcinoma

KAPOSI'S SARCOMA (KS)

Clinical features
1. Affects one-third of patients with AIDS
2. Lesions can be cutaneous or mucosal
3. Approximately 35% occur in the head and neck region, the palate being the most common site
4. Rarely fatal.

ORAL LEUCOPLAKIA

Clinical features
1. Affects lateral border or ventral surface of tongue
2. Spontaneous regression and recurrence common
3. Biopsy should be reserved for persistant or progressive cases
4. Characteristic histological appearance ('Hairy Leucoplakia')

CANDIDIASIS

Clinical features
1. Can involve oral cavity, pharynx or oesophagus
2. Oesophageal involvement associated with
   - (i) Severe dysphagia
   - (ii) Cobblestone appearance of Ba swallow
   - (iii) Stricture formation

Index